Review and Resource Manual

Nursing Case Management

4th Edition

CONTINUING EDUCATION SOURCE

NURSING CERTIFICATION REVIEW MANUAL

CLINICAL PRACTICE RESOURCE

Margaret Leonard, MS, RN-BC, FNP
Elaine Miller, MSN, RN-BC

NURSING
KNOWLEDGE
CENTER

Library of Congress Cataloging-in-Publication Data

Leonard, Margaret.
    Nursing case management review and resource manual. – 4th ed. / by Margaret Leonard, Elaine A. Miller.
    p. ; cm.
    Rev. ed. of: Case management review and resource manual / Anne Llewellyn and Margaret Leonard. 3rd ed. 2009.
    Includes bibliographical references and index.
    ISBN 9781935213383 (alk. paper)
I. Miller, Elaine A. II. Llewellyn, Anne. Nursing case management review and resource manual. III. American Nurses Credentialing Center.
IV. Title.
    [DNLM: 1. Case Management–Nurses' Instruction. 2. Delivery of Health Care–Nurses' Instruction. 3. Professional Competence–Nurses' Instruction. W 84.7]

    362.11068–dc23

                        2012040334

The American Nurses Credentialing Center (ANCC), a subsidiary of the American Nurses Association (ANA), provides individuals and organizations throughout the nursing profession with the resources they need to achieve practice excellence. ANCC's internationally renowned credentialing programs certify nurses in specialty practice areas; recognize healthcare organizations for promoting safe, positive work environments through the Magnet Recognition Program® and the Pathway to Excellence ® Program; and accredit providers of continuing nursing education. In addition, ANCC's Institute for Credentialing Innovation provides leading-edge information and education services and products to support its core credentialing programs.

ISBN 13: 9781935213383

© 2012 American Nurses Credentialing Center.
8515 Georgia Ave., Suite 400
Silver Spring, MD 20910
All rights reserved. Printed with permission.

NURSING CASE MANAGEMENT REVIEW AND RESOURCE MANUAL, 4TH EDITION

NOVEMBER 2012

Please direct your comments and/or queries to: revmanuals@ana.org

The healthcare services delivery system is a volatile marketplace demanding superior knowledge, clinical skills, and competencies from all registered nurses. Nursing autonomy of practice and nurse career marketability and mobility in the new century hinge on affirming the profession's formative philosophy, which places a priority on a lifelong commitment to the principles of education and professional development. The knowledge base of nursing theory and practice is expanding, and while care has been taken to ensure the accuracy and timeliness of the information presented in the **Nursing Case Management Review and Resource Manual**, clinicians are advised to always verify the most current national guidelines and recommendations and to practice in accordance with professional standards of care used with regard to the unique circumstances that apply in each practice situation. In addition, every effort has been made in this text to ensure accuracy and, in particular, to confirm that drug selections and dosages are in accordance with current recommendations and practice, including the ongoing research, changes to government regulations, and the developments in product information provided by pharmaceutical manufacturers. However, it is the responsibility of each nurse practitioner to verify drug product information and to practice in accordance with professional standards of care. In addition, the editors wish to note that provision of information in this text does not imply an endorsement of any particular products, procedures or services.

Therefore, the authors, editors, American Nurses Association (ANA), American Nurses Association's Publishing (ANP), American Nurses Credentialing Center (ANCC), and the Nursing Knowledge Center cannot accept responsibility for errors or omissions, or for any consequences or liability, injury, and/or damages to persons or property from application of the information in this manual and make no warranty, express or implied, with respect to the contents of the **Nursing Case Management Review and Resource Manual**. Completion of this manual does not guarantee that the reader will pass the certification exam. The practice examination questions are not a requirement to take a certification examination. The practice examination questions cannot be used as an indicator of results on the actual certification.

PUBLISHED BY
Nursing Knowledge Center
8515 Georgia Avenue, Suite 400
Silver Spring, MD 20910-3402
www.nursingknowledgecenter.org

NURSING CASE MANAGEMENT REVIEW AND RESOURCE MANUAL, 4TH EDITION

NOVEMBER 2012

Please direct your comments and/or queries to: revmanuals@ana.org

The healthcare services delivery system is a volatile marketplace demanding superior knowledge, clinical skills, and competencies from all registered nurses. Nursing autonomy of practice and nurse career marketability and mobility in the new century hinge on affirming the profession's formative philosophy which places a priority on a lifelong commitment to the principles of education and professional development. The knowledge base of nursing theory and practice is expanding, and while care has been taken to ensure the accuracy and completeness of the information presented in the Nursing Case Management Review and Resource Manual, clinicians are advised to always verify the most current national guidelines, recommendations, and to practice in accordance with professional standards of care used with regard to the unique circumstances that apply in each practice situation. In addition, every effort has been made in this text to ensure accuracy and, in particular, to confirm that drug selections and dosages are in accordance with current recommendations and practice, including the ongoing research, changes to government regulations, and the development in product information provided by pharmaceutical manufacturers. However, it is the responsibility of each nurse practitioner to verify drug product information and to practice in accordance with professional standards of care. In addition, the editors wish to note that provision of information in this text does not imply an endorsement of any particular products, procedures, or services.

Therefore, the authors, editors, American Nurses Association (ANA), American Nurses Association's Publishing (ANP), American Nurses Credentialing Center (ANCC), and the Nursing Knowledge Center cannot accept responsibility for errors or omissions, or for any consequences or liability, injury and/or damages to persons or property from application of the information in this manual and make no warranty, express or implied, with respect to the contents of the Nursing Case Management Review and Resource Manual. Completion of this manual does not guarantee that the reader will pass the certification exam. The practice examination questions are not a requirement to take a certification examination. The practice examination questions cannot be used as an indicator of results on the actual certification.

PUBLISHED BY
Nursing Knowledge Center
8515 Georgia Avenue, Suite 400
Silver Spring, MD 20910-3492
www.nursingknowledgecenter.org

INTRODUCTION TO THE CONTINUING EDUCATION (CE) CONTACT HOUR APPLICATION PROCESS FOR *NURSING CASE MANAGEMENT REVIEW AND RESOURCE MANUAL, 4TH EDITION*

The American Nurses Credentialing Center offers continuing nursing education contact hours (CE) for review and study of this manual. To obtain CE credit you must purchase and complete your review of the manual, pay required fees to enroll in the online module, and complete all module components by the published CE expiration date including disclosures, pre- and post-tests, and the course evaluation. The continuing nursing education contact hours online module can be completed at any time prior to the published CE expiration date and a certificate can be printed from the online learning management system immediately after successful completion of the online module.

For successful completion of the online module, a nurse can receive continuing education contact hours. For more information about the earning CE for this manual visit the list of manual publications on Nursing Knowledge Center's website **www.nursingknowledgecenter.org/Education.**

Inquiries or Comments

If you have any questions about the content of the manual please **e-mail revmanuals@ana.org.** If you have questions about the CE credit offered for review and study of the manual please **e-mail ananursece@ana.org.** You may also mail any comments to Editorial Project Manager at the address listed below.

Nursing Knowledge Center
Attn: Editorial Project Manager
8515 Georgia Avenue, Suite 400
Silver Spring, MD 20910-3492
Fax: (301) 628-5342

CE Provider Information

ANA's Center for Continuing Education and Professional Development is accredited as a provider of continuing nursing education by the American Nurses Credentialing Center's Commission on Accreditation.

ANCC Provider Number 0023.

ANA is approved by the California Board of Registered Nursing, Provider Number CEP6178.

ACKNOWLEDGEMENTS

The authors gratefully acknowledge the foundational work provided by Anne Llewellyn, MS, RN-BC, BSHA, CCM, CRRN, on the previous edition of this manual.

CONTENTS

CHAPTER 1

TAKING THE CERTIFICATION EXAMINATION

When you sign up to take a national certification exam, you will be instructed to go online and review the testing and renewal handbook (www.nursecredentialing.org/documents/certification/application/generaltestingandrenewalhandbook.aspx). Review it carefully and be sure to bookmark the site so you can refer to it frequently. It contains information on test content and sample questions. This is critical information; it will give you insight into the nature of the test. The agency will send you information about the test site; keep this in a safe place until needed.

GENERAL SUGGESTIONS FOR PREPARING FOR THE EXAM

Step One: Control Your Anxiety

Everyone experiences anxiety when faced with taking the certification exam.

- ▶ Remember, your program was designed to prepare you to take this exam.
- ▶ Your instructors took a similar exam, and have probably talked to students who took exams more recently, so they know how to help you prepare.
- ▶ Taking a review course or setting up your own study plan will help you feel more confident about taking the exam.

Step Two: Do Not Listen to Gossip About the Exam

A large volume of information exists about the tests based on reports from people who have taken the exams in the past. Because information from the testing facilities is limited, it is hard to ignore this gossip.

▶ Remember that gossip about the exam that you hear from others is not verifiable.

▶ Because this gossip is based on the imperfect memory of people in a stressful situation, it may not be very accurate.

▶ People tend to remember those items testing content with which they are less comfortable; for instance, those with a limited background in women's health may say that the exam was "all women's health." In fact, the exam blueprint ensures that the exam covers multiple content areas without overemphasizing any one.

Step Three: Set Reasonable Expectations for Yourself

▶ Do not expect to know everything.

▶ Do not try to know everything in great detail.

▶ You do not need a perfect score to pass the exam.

▶ The exam is designed for a beginner level—it is testing readiness for *entry-level* practice.

▶ Learn the general rules, not the exceptions.

▶ The most likely diagnoses will be on the exam, not questions on rare diseases or atypical cases.

▶ Think about the most likely presentation and most common therapy.

Step Four: Prepare Mentally and Physically

▶ While you are getting ready to take the exam, take good physical care of yourself.

▶ Get plenty of sleep and exercise, and eat well while preparing for the exam.

▶ These things are especially important while you are studying and immediately before you take the exam.

Step Five: Access Current Knowledge

General Content

You will be given a list of general topics that will be on the exam when you register to take the exam. In addition, examine the table of contents of this book and the test content outline, available at www.nursecredentialing.org/cert/TCOs.html.

▶ What content do you need to know?

▶ How well do you know these subjects?

Take a Review Course

▶ Taking a review course is an excellent way to assess your knowledge of the content that will be included in the exam.

▶ If you plan to take a review course, take it well before the exam so you will have plenty of time to master any areas of weakness the course uncovers.

▶ If you are prepared for the exam, you will not hear anything new in the course. You will be familiar with everything that is taught.

▶ If some topics in the review course are new to you, concentrate on these in your studies.

▶ People have a tendency to study what they know; it is rewarding to study something and feel a mastery of it! Unfortunately, this will not help you master unfamiliar content. Be sure to use a review course to identify your areas of strength and weakness, then concentrate on the weaknesses.

Depth of Knowledge

▶ How much do you need to know about a subject?

▶ You cannot know everything about a topic.

▶ Study the information sent to you from the testing agency, what you were taught in school, what is covered in this text, and the general guidelines given in this chapter.

▶ Look at practice tests designed for the exam. Practice tests for other exams will not be helpful.

▶ Consult your class notes or clinical diagnosis and management textbook for the major points about a disease. Additional reference books can be found online at www.nursecredentialing.org/cert/refs.html.

▶ For example, with regard to medications, know the drug categories and the major medications in each. Assume all drugs in a category are generally alike, and then focus on the differences among common drugs. Know the most important indications, contraindications, and side effects. Emphasize safety. The questions usually do not require you to know the exact dosage of a drug.

Step Six: Institute a Systematic Study Plan

Develop Your Study Plan

▶ Write up a formal plan of study.

  ▸ Include topics for study, timetable, resources, and methods of study that work for you.

  ▸ Decide whether you want to organize a study group or work alone.

  ▸ Schedule regular times to study.

  ▸ Avoid cramming; it is counterproductive. Try to schedule your study periods in 1-hour increments.

▶ Identify resources to use for studying. To prepare for the examination, you should have the following materials on your shelf:

  ▸ This review book.

  ▸ Your class notes.

  ▸ Other important sources, including: information from the testing facility, a clinical diagnosis textbook, favorite journal articles, notes from a review course, and practice tests.

  ▸ Consult the bibliography on the test blueprint. When studying less familiar material, it is helpful to study using the same references that the testing center uses.

▶ You will need to know facts and be able to interpret and analyze this information utilizing critical thinking.

Personalize Your Study Plan

▶ How do you learn best?

  ▸ If you learn best by listening or talking, attend a review course or discuss topics with a colleague.

▶ Read everything the test facility sends you as soon as you receive it and several times during your preparation period. It will give you valuable information to help guide your study.

▶ Have a specific place with good lighting set aside for studying. Find a quiet place with no distractions. Assemble your study materials.

Implement Your Study Plan

You must have basic content knowledge. In addition, you must be able to use this information to think critically and make decisions based on facts.

- ▶ Refer to your study plan regularly.

- ▶ Stick to your schedule.

- ▶ Take breaks when you get tired.

- ▶ If you start procrastinating, get help from a friend or reorganize your study plan.

- ▶ It is not necessary to follow your plan rigidly. Adjust as you learn where you need to spend more time.

- ▶ Memorize the basics of the content areas you will be required to know.

Focus on General Material

- ▶ Most of what you need to know is basic material that does not require constant updating.

- ▶ You do not need to worry about the latest information being published as you are studying for the exam. Remember, it can take 6 to 12 months for new information to be incorporated into test questions.

Pace Your Studying

- ▶ Stop studying for the examination when you are starting to feel overwhelmed and look at what is bothering you. Then make changes.

- ▶ Break overwhelming tasks into smaller tasks that you know you can do.

- ▶ Stop and take breaks while studying.

Work With Others

- ▶ Talk with classmates about your preparation for the exam.

- ▶ Keep in touch with classmates, and help each other stick to your study plans.

- ▶ If your classmates become anxious, do not let their anxiety affect you. Walk away if you need to.

- ▶ Do not believe bad stories you hear about other people's experiences with previous exams.

- ▶ Remember, you know as much as anyone about what will be on the next exam!

Consider a Study Group

- ▶ Study groups can provide practice in analyzing cases, interpreting questions, and critical thinking.

    - You can discuss a topic and take turns presenting cases for the group to analyze.

    - Study groups can also provide moral support and help you continue studying.

Step Seven: Strategies Immediately Before the Exam

Final Preparation Suggestions

▶ Use practice exams when studying to get accustomed to the exam format and time restrictions.

- Many books that are labeled as review books are simply a collection of examination questions.

- If you have test anxiety, such practice tests may help alleviate the anxiety.

- Practice tests can help you learn to judge the time it should take you to complete the exam.

- Practice tests are useful for gaining experience in analyzing questions.

- Books of questions may not uncover the gaps in your knowledge that a more systematic content review text will reveal.

- If you feel that you don't know enough about a topic, refer to a text to learn more. After you feel that you have learned the topic, practice questions are a wonderful tool to help improve your test-taking skill.

▶ Know your test-taking style.

- Do you rush through the exam without reading the questions thoroughly?

- Do you get stuck and dwell on a question for a long time?

- You should spend about 45 to 60 seconds per question and finish with time to review the questions you were not sure about.

- Be sure to read the question completely, including all four answer choices. Choice "a" may be good, but "d" may be best.

The Night Before the Exam

▶ Be prepared to get to the exam on time.

- Know the test site location and how long it takes to get there.

- Take a "dry run" beforehand to make sure you know how to get to the testing site, if necessary.

- Get a good night's sleep.

- Eat sensibly.

- Avoid alcohol the night before.

- Assemble the required material—two forms of identification and watch. Both IDs must match the name on the application, and one photo ID is preferred.

- Know the exam room rules.

  ▷ You will be given scratch paper, which will be collected at the end of the exam.

  ▷ Nothing else is allowed in the exam room.

  ▷ You will be required to put papers, backpacks, etc., in a corner of the room or in a locker.

▷ No water or food will be allowed.

▷ You will be allowed to walk to a water fountain and go to the bathroom one at a time.

The Day of the Exam

▶ Get there early. You must arrive to the test center at least 15 minutes before your scheduled appointment time. If you are late, you may not be admitted.

▶ Think positively. You have studied hard and are well-prepared.

▶ Remember your anxiety reduction strategies.

Specific Tips for Dealing With Anxiety

Test anxiety is a specific type of anxiety. Symptoms include upset stomach, sweaty palms, tachycardia, trouble concentrating, and a feeling of dread. But there are ways to cope with test anxiety.

▶ There is no substitute for being well-prepared.

▶ Practice relaxation techniques.

▶ Avoid alcohol, excess coffee, caffeine, and any new medications that might sedate you, dull your senses, or make you feel agitated.

▶ Take a few deep breaths and concentrate on the task at hand.

Focus on Specific Test-Taking Skills

To do well on the exam, you need good test-taking skills in addition to knowledge of the content and ability to use critical thinking.

All Certification Exams Are Multiple Choice

▶ Multiple-choice tests have specific rules for test construction.

▶ A multiple-choice question consists of three parts: the information (or stem), the question, and the four possible answers (one correct and three distracters).

▶ Careful analysis of each part is necessary. Read the entire question before answering.

▶ Practice your test-taking skills by analyzing the practice questions in this book and on the ANCC Web site.

Analyze the Information Given

▶ Do not assume you have more information than is given.

▶ Do not overanalyze.

▶ Remember, the writer of the question assumes this is all of the information needed to answer the question.

▶ If information is not given, it is not relevant and will not affect the answer.

▶ Do not make the question more complicated than it is.

What Kind of Question Is Asked?

▶ Are you supposed to recall a fact, apply facts to a situation, or understand and differentiate between options?

    ▸ Read the question thinking about what the writer is asking.

    ▸ Look for key words or phrases that lead you (see Figure 1–1). These help determine what kind of answer the question requires.

FIGURE 1–1.
EXAMPLES OF KEY WORDS AND PHRASES

▶ avoid	▶ initial	▶ most
▶ best	▶ first	▶ significant
▶ except	▶ contributing to	▶ likely
▶ not	▶ appropriate	▶ of the following
		▶ most consistent with

Read All of the Answers

▶ If you are absolutely certain that answer "a" is correct as you read it, mark it, but read the rest of the question so you do not trick yourself into missing a better answer.

▶ If you are absolutely sure answer "a" is wrong, cross it off or make a note on your scratch paper and continue reading the question.

▶ After reading the entire question, go back, analyze the question, and select the best answer.

▶ Do not jump ahead.

▶ If the question asks you for an assessment, the best answer will be an assessment. Do not be distracted by an intervention that sounds appropriate.

▶ If the question asks you for an intervention, do not answer with an assessment.

▶ When two answer choices sound very good, the best one is usually the least expensive, least invasive way to achieve the goal. For example, if your answer choices include a physical exam maneuver or imaging, the physical exam maneuver is probably the better choice provided it will give the information needed.

▶ If the answers include two options that are the opposite of each other, one of the two is probably the correct answer.

▶ When numeric answers cover a wide range, a number in the middle is more likely to be correct.

▶ Watch out for distracters that are correct but do not answer the question, combine true and false information, or contain a word or phrase that is similar to the correct answer.

▶ Err on the side of caution.

Only One Answer Can Be Correct

▶ When more than one suggested answer is correct, you must identify the one that best answers the question asked.

▶ If you cannot choose between two answers, you have a 50% chance of getting it right if you guess.

Avoid Changing Answers

▶ Change an answer only if you have a compelling reason, such as you remembered something additional, or you understand the question better after rereading it.

▶ People change to a wrong answer more often than to a right answer.

Time Yourself to Complete the Whole Exam

▶ Do not spend a large amount of time on one question.

▶ If you cannot answer a question quickly, mark it and continue the exam.

▶ If time is left at the end, return to the difficult questions.

▶ Make educated guesses by eliminating the obviously wrong answers and choosing a likely answer even if you are not certain.

▶ Trust your instinct.

▶ Answer every question. There is no penalty for a wrong answer.

▶ Occasionally a question will remind you of something that helps you with a question earlier in the test. Look back at that question to see if what you are remembering affects how you would answer that question.

ABOUT THE CERTIFICATION EXAMS

The American Nurses Credentialing Center Computerized Exam

The ANCC examination is given only as a computer exam, and each exam is different.

The order of the questions is scrambled for every test, so even if two people are taking the same exam, the questions will be in a different order. The exam consists of 175 multiple-choice questions.

▶ 150 of the 175 questions are part of the test and how you answer will count toward your score; 25 are included to refine questions and will not be scored. You will not know which ones count, so treat all questions the same.

▶ You will need to know how to use a mouse, scroll by either clicking arrows on the scroll bar or using the up and down arrow keys, and perform other basic computer tasks.

▶ The exam does not require computer expertise.

▶ However, if you are not comfortable with using a computer, you should practice using a mouse and computer beforehand so you do not waste time on the mechanics of using the computer.

Know What to Expect During the Test

▶ Each ANCC test question is independent of the other questions.

  ▸ For each case study, there is only one question. This means that a correct answer on any question does not depend on the correct answer to any other question.

  ▸ Each question has four possible answers. There are no questions asking for combinations of correct answers (such as "a and c") or multiple-multiples.

▶ You can skip a question and go back to it at the end of the exam.

▶ You cannot mark key words in the question or right or wrong answers. If you want to do this, use the scratch paper.

▶ You will get your results immediately, and a grade report will be provided upon leaving the testing site.

Internet Resources

▶ ANCC Web site: www.nursecredentialing.org

▶ ANA Bookstore: www.nursesbooks.org. Catalog of ANA nursing scope and standards publications and other titles that may be listed on your test content outline

▶ National Guideline Clearinghouse: www.ngc.gov

CHAPTER 2

CLINICAL CASE MANAGEMENT PRACTICE

> **"**I think one's feelings waste themselves in words; they ought all to be distilled into actions which bring results.**"**
> —*Florence Nightingale*

Case managers focus on care coordination, financial management, and resource utilization to yield cost-effective outcomes that are patient-centric, safe, and provided in the least restrictive setting. When case management is practiced in this manner, costs are contained and patients, families, and stakeholders are viewed as essential members of the team. Case management is a fluid and dynamic practice that is most effective when it changes and adapts with the challenges of the healthcare system. Stewardship of the healthcare dollars, safe transitions of care, evaluating patient adherence, and consistent stakeholder communication are critical interventions that case managers employ, while maintaining a primary and consistent focus on quality of care and patient self-determination.

Case management is not a new concept. It traces its history back to the early 1900s, when it simply functioned as a means of providing care and containing healthcare costs. In the 1920s, the practice found its roots in the fields of psychiatry and social work, and focused on long-term chronic illnesses that were managed within the community. Case management processes were also used by visiting and public health nurses in the 1930s, when making house calls was a common practice. Throughout the next 50 years, case management remained essentially in the community. The mid-1980s saw the introduction of prospective payment system (PPS) case management, which became widespread within the acute and post-acute settings (Cesta, Tahan, & Fink, 2002). Case managers are found across the continuum of care and serve as advocates for patients and their families navigating the complex healthcare system. Their multifaceted roles ensure that patients receive high-quality care in the least restrictive settings for the most cost-effective price in an organized and coordinated manner. Today, case managers are the vital link in a complex healthcare system that is often unfamiliar and confusing.

The practice of case management is designed to formulate a plan that enables the patient to move smoothly through the healthcare system. To achieve this, case managers work closely with many stakeholders: patients, their family members, their caregivers, the healthcare team, payers, and communites.

Case management is not a profession unto itself but a practice that encompasses many disciplines. Nursing is the predominant field of the practice of case management, while social workers and other healthcare professionals combine to make up a mix of dynamic professionals with a central goal—to focus the system and facilitate the delivery of care. The discipline of nursing focuses on the whole person, which is a key case management concept. The broad training and skills that nurses acquire allow them to assess patients' needs and work collaboratively with all involved in their patients' care. It is important to remember that no single discipline owns the practice of case management. Therefore, it is essential that each individual involved in the practice follow his or her governing state's Practice Act as dictated by his or her respective discipline.

Case Simulation: A nurse case manager, working telephonically with a patient located in another state, is aware of the Nurse Practice Act in his or her state as well as the Nurse Practice Act for the state in which the patient is located.

NURSING CASE MANAGEMENT CONCEPTS

Definitions

Many of the leading professional organizations have adopted definitions of case management, including the National Association of Social Workers (NASW), the American Board for Occupational Health Nurses (ABOHN), and the Association of Rehabilitation Nurses (ARN). Each definition is slightly different, but similar in context. As the practice of case management continues to mature, one definition uniting the practice will hopefully evolve. Until that time, the following are two descriptions used to define the practice of case management.

The approved definition of nursing case management by the American Nurses Credentialing Center (ANCC) states:

> Nursing Case Management is a dynamic and systematic collaborative approach to providing and coordinating healthcare services to a defined population. It is a participative process to identify and facilitate options and services for meeting individuals' health needs, while decreasing fragmentation and duplication of care, and enhancing quality, cost-effective clinical outcomes. The framework for nursing case management includes five components: assessment, planning, implementation, evaluation, and interaction. (Llewelyn & Leonard, 2009, p. 12)

The Case Management Society of America (CMSA) supports a multidisciplinary role for case management, rather than focusing on case management as a function of one specific discipline. The definition of case management, updated in 2010 and published in the CMSA's *Standards of Practice for Case Management,* is:

> Case management is a collaborative process of assessment, planning, facilitation, care coordination, evaluation and advocacy for options and services to meet an individual's and family's comprehensive health needs through communication and available resources to promote quality cost-effective outcomes. (CMSA, 2010, p. 8)

> The philosophy of case management is that all individuals are eligible for case management services regardless of age, culture, or ability to pay for service. Yet, it is important to realize that not everyone requires case management. Applying an accepted business principle—the Pareto principle or the 80/20 rule—to health care, it is estimated that 80% of all healthcare resources are utilized by 20% of the population. This rule basically states that 80% of the "outcomes" come from 20% of the "inputs." (McDonough, 2011)

This ratio reveals the population most appropriate for case management services. For case management to succeed, early risk identification, using proven indicators, and the stratification of the group according to these indicators is critical so that appropriate interventions and resources are utilized.

Case management is a voluntary service, so gaining permission from, and establishing trust with the patient, family, and caregivers is critical. To achieve positive outcomes, the cooperation of the patient, family, and caregiver is needed to ensure adherence with the plan of care. Today, a key aspect of effective nursing case management is the ability to assess an individual's knowledge, motivation, and attitude toward care in order to influence adherence.

NURSING CASE MANAGEMENT CONCEPTS: ROLES AND FUNCTIONS

The nurse case manager's clinical expertise and holistic approach are the vital connections between the individual patient, the provider, the payer, and the community (see Figure 2–1). Clinical expertise and integrated care management are vital connections between stakeholders: patient, family, and caregiver; interdisciplinary team; payers; and communities. Those who enter the practice need to demonstrate competency in many areas. The Case Management Society of America's *Standards of Practice* describe them as:

▶ "Assessment of health and psychosocial needs, including health literacy, and development of a case management plan collaboratively with all stakeholders

▶ Planning with all stakeholders to maximize healthcare responses, quality, and cost-effective outcomes

▶ Facilitating communication and coordination among stakeholders, involving the patient in the decision-making process in order to minimize service fragmentation

▶ Educating the patient and all stakeholders on treatment options, community resources, insurance benefits, and psychosocial concerns so that timely and informed decisions can be made

▶ Empowering the patient to problem solve by exploring care options and alternative plans, when necessary, to achieve desired outcome

▶ Encouraging the appropriate use of healthcare services and striving to improve the quality of care and maintain cost-effectiveness on a case-by-case basis

▶ Assisting the client in safe transitions of care to the next most appropriate level

▶ Striving to promote patient self-advocacy and self-determination

▶ Advocating for both the patient and stakeholders, to facilitate positive outcomes. However, if a conflict arises, the patient must be the priority." (CMSA, 2010)

It is essential that the nurse case manager be astute in the nursing process and acquire keen assessment skills, be clinically competent, and be able to identify patients at risk and their actual and potential health problems. The role of change agent is vital for a nurse case manager because planning, facilitating, and collaborating on a plan of care may require all the involved parties to be open to many possibilities. The nurse case manager's leadership abilities ensure that the healthcare team works collaboratively in meeting the needs of the patient, family, and caregivers. Proactively monitoring responses to care and treatment, and recommending changes to the plan of care, are critical to produce effective outcomes. Finally, excellent communication skills must be employed to articulate the case management plan and expected outcomes.

FIGURE 2–1.
HEALTHCARE TEAM

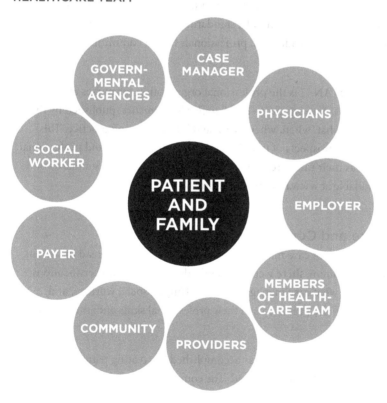

Standards of Practice

Each profession establishes its own standards of practice. Members of these professions—the professionals—are assumed to have extensive theoretical knowledge and possess skills based on knowledge that they are able to apply in practice. Members of professions organize professional bodies, which are intended to enhance the status of their membership and have carefully controlled entrance requirements. Professions have extensive periods of education and testing for competence. Before being admitted to membership of a professional body, there is usually a requirement to pass prescribed examinations based on theoretical knowledge. In addition to examinations, there is usually a requirement for periods of institutionalized training where aspiring professionals acquire specified practical experience in a trainee role before being recognized as a full member of the professional body. Mandatory continuing education, through professional development, updates the professional's skills and knowledge. Licensed practitioners have a code of professional conduct, or ethics, and disciplinary actions are taken for those who infringe upon the code.

Professions are self-regulating and independent from government. They tend to be policed and regulated by senior, respected practitioners and the most highly qualified members of the profession. Professionals are autonomous and mobile; standardization of professional training and procedures enhances this mobility. In addition, professionals have a commitment to public service and altruism.

The American Nurses Association (ANA) is the professional organization for nurses and sets the standards of practice for nurses. *Nursing: Scope and Standards of Practice*, published by the ANA (2010), articulates the who, what, when, where, why, and how of nursing practice. This document discusses the scope and prospects of practice and delineates practice and professional performance standards as well as their measurement criteria. There are 16 ANA Standards of Practice; this document is available at www.nursingworld.org.

Professional Excellence and Competence

In the early 1980s, when the practice of case management was becoming widespread in various settings throughout the care continuum, there were no standards of practice, no certifications, and no formal policies explaining what case management was. Nurses, social workers, and vocational specialists who made up the practice used their professional skills and intuition to find their way instead.

Those early pioneers said that case management was accomplished by treating patients in the same ways they would want their families to be treated. The competencies of this "Golden Rule," that is, "do unto others," included clinical experience, compassion, empathy, personal relationship skills, and common sense. The goal was then as it is now—to ensure that patients received safe care, at the right time, in the right place, and for the most cost-effective price.

In 1990, those early leaders formed the Case Management Society of America (CMSA). CMSA is dedicated to the support and development of case management practice through educational forums, networking opportunities, and legislative involvement. Unique in its composition as an international organization, CMSA's success and strength is its structure as a member-driven society (CMSA, 2012).

Case management leaders began to explore how one could validate one's expertise. By networking with the organizations that provided certifications in the areas of disability management and vocational care, the group set up the first certification for case managers and developed both the exam and the established criteria by which professionals would be measured in order to determine whether they were qualified to sit for the examination. The first certification examination was given in 1993 by the Commission for Case Management Certification. Since that time, other certifying bodies have established case management certification examinations. Organizations, such as the American Nurses Credentialing Center and others, challenge nurses who are engaged in the practice of case management to test their knowledge. As a result of the process of certification, the practice of case management has gained credibility throughout the healthcare industry and among employers, practitioners, government officials, the military healthcare system, consumers, payers, and other stakeholders.

In 1995, CMSA was the first organization to develop the *Standards of Practice*. The standards allowed those in the practice to demonstrate to physicians, payers, legislators, and other members of the healthcare team exactly what the practice of case management was about (CMSA, 2010). The case management *Standards of Practice* make it possible for hospitals, managed care organizations, and independent case managers to build policies and procedures that ensure their organizations are compliant with the requirements established by licensing bodies and accreditation organizations.

With standards of practice in place and a credential to validate professionals in the practice, case management has spread throughout every aspect of the healthcare system. In order to sustain the practice, organizations recruit professionals into the field from various disciplines. As a result, training programs needed to educate those coming from various clinical settings on their roles as case managers have evolved.

Case management is a multidisciplinary practice, yet the majority of practicing case managers are nurses. The initial training of those new to the practice includes the history of the practice, introduction to the case management *Standards of Practice*, and an overview of the job description and training in the organization's policies and procedures. In addition, a new case manager needs to be familiar with the *Code of Professional Conduct*, as well as the laws and regulatory statutes that affect case management practice. The orientation, continuing education, and staff training allows professionals with diverse clinical expertise to unite under the case management umbrella and forge a common bond, while still maintaining their individual professional identities.

Preceptorship and Mentorship

The core components of the practice of case management are the same across all settings. Yet each setting has its own rules and regulatory issues that case managers must be aware of and follow. For example, case managers who practice in the hospital setting come in contact with a variety of payers' policies, regulations, and legislation to which they must adhere. Those who work in managed care organizations must be aware of the various benefits plans offered and the regulations that accompany these plans in the states where they are offered. Those in workers' compensation must follow the specific laws and regulations set forth by each state. To ensure case management professionals understand the nuances of their practice, organization policies and procedures, and are trained and informed, preceptorship and mentoring programs are an integral part of most orientation programs.

Mentoring and preceptorship programs are two of the more commonly used role-modeling programs designed to sustain the learning and professional growth of nurses and to promote the overall quality of the practice settings. Many aspects of mentoring and preceptorship are similar. Both approaches depend upon effective one-on-one role-modeling; self-directed learning; a safe environment for reflection and practice; and the acts of advising, counseling, guiding, advocating, recognizing strengths, and providing constructive feedback (*Advanced Mentoring Healthcare*, 2008).

Preceptors offer staff development, training, technical assistance, and quality control through the development of an individualized tutorial relationship with each case manager. It is a unique program of professional growth and development designed for each case manager being supervised. Preceptors are generally experienced case managers who provide support and guidance to new members of the team. Preceptors work closely with students ("preceptees") on an ongoing basis to plan the orientation and to review clinical practice and learning experiences that may arise. This enhances the preceptee's awareness of various scenarios while the preceptor monitors the preceptee's progress and provides feedback on performance in order to help with the transition and integration into the organization. Preceptorships tend to focus on a formal process for helping the new professional acquire beginning-practice competencies through direct supervision over a limited period of time.

Mentoring is either informal or formal and usually focuses on broader learning and career development, as well as personal and professional growth, through a consultative approach over a longer time. Professionals may engage in several mentoring experiences over their professional careers. The length of the relationship ranges from months to years and is determined by the time required for the mentee to achieve his or her objectives. A mentoring relationship differs from preceptorship because it is

▶ Less instructional,

▶ Focused less on supervision and assessment of performance, and

▶ Focused more on positively influencing behavior through role-modeling and guidance.

Functions of good mentors include

▶ Demonstrating role expertise and promoting role socialization;

▶ Providing a vision by role-modeling and offering direction for career development;

▶ Providing a reflective practice that enables the mentee to determine how and why decisions are made and how these decisions influence positive outcomes;

▶ Sharing values and customs;

▶ Providing support and structure, which involves listening, befriending the mentee, expressing positive expectations, and helping the mentee to make the experience rewarding;

▶ Setting high standards and demanding a high level of performance;

▶ Empowering the mentee to reach autonomy that comes from competency, self-confidence, and responsibility; and

▶ Opening doors and facilitating important contacts through networking (Busen & Engebretson, 1999).

To have a robust leadership in the future, senior management must be involved in the mentoring programs of their primary professionals. In addition to mentoring, another approach used to develop leaders is to highlight career ladder programs, with case management as a clinical system management option. Through outreach efforts, today's case managers look for potential leaders to promote. Once identified, these individuals should be supported through

▶ Mentoring relationships,

▶ Leadership skill-building,

▶ Educational programs based on the latest leadership evidence, and

▶ Safe opportunities to hone their skills through volunteer leadership experiences in professional societies and within their own communities and employment settings (Forcible Figures: J. Bowman, 2008).

In the book *The Extraordinary Leader: Turning Good Managers Into Great Leaders*, John H. Zenger and Joseph Folkman (2002) offer the following insight into leadership development: "Good does not equal great—and your organization needs you to be great." Organizations need to invest in identifying strong internal candidates and provide opportunities for them to become extraordinary.

Staff Development

The primary purpose of staff development is to support the learning needs of the professionals who work within an organization by providing opportunities for the acquisition of new knowledge, skills, and behaviors in view of advancing technologies, changing healthcare delivery systems, expanding roles, and case management research. These opportunities include continuing education, formal and informal inservices, coaching, and consulting.

Staff Training Programs

Orientation and ongoing training programs help ensure that staff are kept up-to-date and have the knowledge and resources to provide quality services to those with whom they work. Staff training may vary by profession and organization type. Examples of training include obtaining continuing education credits in a relevant field, attending meetings or conferences related to job functions, and participating in employer-sponsored programs on job function performance and clinical competencies.

Staff training programs include:

▶ Initial orientation or training for all staff before assuming assigned roles and responsibilities

▶ Ongoing training, at a minimum annually, to maintain professional competency

▶ Training in accreditation standards as appropriate to job functions

▶ Training in state and regulatory requirements related to job functions

▶ Training on conflict of interest and confidentiality responsibilities

▶ Training on identification and prevention of fraud and abuse, as appropriate to job functions

▶ Training of staff for work that is delegated and the oversight required according to their job functions

All training should be documented and maintained for licensure bodies, accreditation organizations, and the individual's professional personnel file. For those professionals who are independent, the same standard applies, except that the costs for those activities are paid for by the professional.

Self-Evaluation and Peer Review

To be effective leaders, case management professionals need to have finely tuned skills. These include having up-to-date clinical skills; psychosocial skills in order to be able to recognize and understand barriers to adherence that patients display; business skills to understand the business of health care; and personal skills, such as insight into financial management. They need to be able to communicate the outcomes they achieve to various stakeholders to validate their place as an integral member of the healthcare team. Achieving these skills requires professionals to adopt a mindset that commits them to continual learning. To do this, they need to budget time and dollars to achieve their professional education competencies and goals.

Case managers need to take an active role in their professional development activities. They need to take time to self-evaluate in order to understand gaps in their expertise, and take steps to close those gaps and meet their ongoing professional goals. Results of self-evaluation often result in the motivation that professionals need to go back to school to obtain advanced degrees, learn new skills, move into new positions, or even to change jobs so that they stay fresh and creative.

Most organizations maintain formal assessment programs for individual staff members, such as annual performance appraisals and ongoing audits of their work. The annual performance appraisal is also a good time to review the current status of licensure and certifications, review the status of annual and ongoing continuing education for professional competency, and discuss goals that the professional should consider pursuing as part of the professional development process.

PROFESSIONAL ACTIVITIES

Today, most states and territories require licensed healthcare professionals to take part in mandatory continuing education (CE). States require that licensed professionals obtain a specific number of credits within a specific time frame. In addition, states may require a certain amount of hours devoted to specific topics, such as infection control or HIV/AIDs training, and may mandate continuing education for professionals who work less than a given number of hours per year (Medscape, 2011).

Each professional must be aware of the continuing education requirements for the states in which he or she is licensed. Each professional must keep his or her own records and produce those records if audited. If a licensed professional is audited and is unable to produce the required materials per the states' requirements, penalties and loss of license are possible.

In addition to licensure requirements, certified healthcare professionals must comply with the specific requirements of certifying bodies. Compliance with certification, and recertification, criteria is the nurse case manager's responsibility. Most certifying bodies allow professionals to maintain their certifications by participating in continuing education programs and demonstrating compliance by maintaining certificates of completion within a specific time frame. Professionals have the option to retake a certification examination, but most professionals opt to attain the required continuing education.

Continuing education activities are an important part of each nurse case manager's professional development, and with licensure, most certifications specify what types of programs are acceptable. Case managers can and should attend programs and take courses that are directly related to the practice of care management. This gives professionals a broad choice of the type of continuing education credits they earn to improve their individual practice.

Most people obtain continuing education credits by attending conferences or professional organizations' local, state, and national meetings; or through professional journals, webinars, or other social media. As a result of advances in technology, many time-pressed professionals turn to online CE programs.

Through experience, professionals realize that sharing information is important to the practice of case management. Examples of venues for sharing expertise include writing to professional journals, speaking at conferences, or being part of developing programs that assist others in their professional development.

Experienced case managers can also participate in research projects. Research is the means of enhancing the body of knowledge to elevate the practice of case management to a recognized profession. Case managers who participate in, and contribute to, the field of research as advanced practice professionals ensure that the practice moves forward. As the practice of case management continues to evolve and mature, it is important that those with expertise in the area of research use research methodologies to refine and validate the practice.

Lastly, professional organizations provide important professional growth opportunities for case managers. CMSA is the largest professional organization dedicated to meeting the needs of case managers. It offers a variety of online education and professional development tools, located in the Educational Resource Library and the CMSA Toolbox at www.cmsa.org. The American Nurses Association (www.nursingworld.org) is the professional association for nurses, with the American Nurses Credentialing Center (ANCC), as its certification arm, providing a wealth of information for professionals seeking certification in a variety of specialties. ANCC's Web site is www.nursecredentialing.org.

Professional organizations provide practitioners the opportunity to be a part of a powerful network of case managers who value the practice and work together to advance it. As part of a professional network, case managers are provided with timely and relevant information about the practice that gives them the ability to be up-to-date with current standards, which allows them to practice safely. In addition, participation in professional organizations provides practitioners with a unified voice and the power to advance the practice of case management.

STANDARDS OF CARE

Standards of care provide minimal as well as optimal parameters from which to measure the quality of health care. Each professional group can refer to its own standards as the benchmark for professional performance in the discipline.

Standards of care help with operationalization of patient care processes by providing a baseline for the quality of care delivered to the patient. An example would be a standard that was universally accepted regarding the care of a patient with chest pain. This standard would allow professionals across the country to have an accepted way to systematically treat those patients who suffer from chest pain. Nurse case managers rely on clinical standards or guidelines to ensure that interventions

- ▶ Are based on scientific, sound consistent practice,
- ▶ Optimize the management of limited resources, and
- ▶ Decrease variations in care.

Examples of standards of care are those set by the American Heart Association (www.americanheart.org), American Diabetes Association (www.diabetes.org), and the American Cancer Society (www.cancer.org).

Frequently, standards of care focus on a particular discipline. This gives the professional involved in the treatment a standard by which to practice. (See CMSA, 2010.)

CLINICAL GUIDELINES

Clinical guidelines or clinical practice guidelines are defined as systematically developed statements that assist the practitioner, healthcare team, and patient in making decisions about appropriate health care for specific clinical circumstances. Clinical guidelines or clinical practice guidelines are used in the healthcare industry to ensure that clinical interventions are less variable; are based on sound, consistent practice; and optimize the management of limited resources. The literature tells us that the time lapse between introduction of a new clinical guideline and adoption by practitioners is about 17 years. Therefore, it may become necessary for a case manager to repeatedly remind providers about the guidelines, but guidelines are just that—guidelines. They are not regulations or legislation. They are tools case managers use to improve the quality of care provided while controlling costs. They are evidence-based or practice-based, patient-specific, and user-friendly.

Most professional organizations have developed guidelines for practice and care delivery specific for interests, such as the American Academy of Pediatrics, which has 96 guidelines; American Academy of Allergy Asthma and Immunology; American Academy of Child and Adolescent Psychiatry; National Association of Pediatric Nurse Practitioners; American Academy of Dermatology; American Academy of Family Physicians; American Academy of Pediatric Dentistry; American College of Chest Physicians; American College of Emergency Physicians; and the like. Many of these guidelines detail the disease categories, the clinical scope, the target population, the interventions, the measures, and the desired outcomes.

The U.S. Preventive Services Task Force (USPSTF) is an independent panel of experts in primary care and prevention that systematically reviews the evidence of effectiveness and develops recommendations for clinical preventive services. Sponsored since 1998 by the Agency for Healthcare Research and Quality (AHRQ), the task force is the leading independent panel of private-sector experts in prevention and primary care. Its pocket guide covers all USPSTF recommendations, organized for quick reference and easy searching, from 2002 through 2010 (USPSTF, 2011).

 Most case management and utilization management systems have guidelines and algorithms built into their case management software. Two of the most popular sets of clinical guidelines are Milliman and InterQual, which are clinical decision-making support tools. Further content on these clinical guidelines is discussed in Chapter 3.

Several organizations have developed Web sites that case managers, healthcare professionals, and the general public can access when they need information on clinical guidelines. Case managers can use these sites to gather information that will assist them to more fully understand a patient's diagnosis and treatment options. Examples of these sites are The National Guideline Clearinghouse™ (NGC) and the W. K. Kellogg Health Science Library. NGC is a public resource sponsored by the AHRQ in partnership with the American Medical Association and the American Association of Health Plans. The Web site to access the clearinghouse is www.guideline.gov. The W. K. Kellogg Health Science Library (www.library.dal.ca/kellogg) contains guidelines derived from evidence-based medicine.

CLINICAL PATHWAYS, CARE PRACTICE, AND CARE MAPS

Although closely related to clinical practice guidelines, pathways more directly target the specific process and sequence of care, frequently plotting out the expected course of an illness or procedure with associated prompts for appropriate interventions. Also known as clinical pathways and care maps, pathways are generally multidisciplinary by design and incorporate the responsibilities of physicians and nurses with those of ancillary medical providers, including pharmacists, physical therapists, and social workers. They are comprehensive algorithms designed to manage the care of patients from the time they enter the system until they are returned to their optimal level of functioning (Klainberg, Holzemer, Leonard, & Arnold, 1998). They are regularly developed at the point of care and may, in some cases, incorporate or even replace traditional chart documentation. In addition, pathways are often evidence-based and may even be integrated with locally or nationally developed clinical practice guidelines. Most pathways, however, are locally developed and are most frequently implemented at the level of the hospital or medical center as part of a cost-containment or quality-assurance initiative.

Clinical pathways are structured, multidisciplinary plans of care designed to support the implementation of clinical guidelines and protocols. They are designed to support clinical management, clinical and nonclinical resource management, clinical audit, and financial management. They provide detailed guidance for each stage in the management of a patient with a specific condition over a given time period, and include progress and outcome details.

Clinical pathways aim to improve the continuity and coordination of care across different disciplines and service lines. They can be viewed as algorithms in as much as they offer a flow chart format of the decisions to be made and the care to be provided for a given patient or patient group for a given condition in a stepwise sequence.

Clinical pathways have four main components: a time line, the categories of care or activities and their interventions, intermediate and long-term outcome criteria, and variance tracking.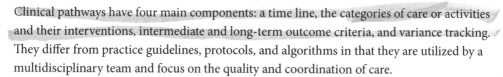 They differ from practice guidelines, protocols, and algorithms in that they are utilized by a multidisciplinary team and focus on the quality and coordination of care.

The case manager uses these tools as a way to proactively identify problems, determine where the problems arose, and gather data that objectively provide information on how improvements to care or processes can be made. The case manager objectively sees how the patient is doing as a result of the use of clinical pathways, since the case manager has a broad view of the process. The case manager does this by continually assessing whether the patient is meeting the expected goals of the pathway. If goals are not achieved, the case manager documents this as a variance.

Variance

Variances can occur at any time throughout the course of treatment. Variances occur when the patient does not progress as outlined according to the clinical pathway. Further discussion on variance tracking is found in Chapter 4. Variances are usually classified according to who or what caused the variance—the patient, individual clinical or healthcare professionals, or a fault in the system. When variances to the clinical pathway occur, documentation shows that the variance occurred and what was done to correct the variance. If variances are a result of complex causes, an interdisciplinary case consultation can convene to discuss the events. The meeting focuses on determining whether the pathway is realistic for the individual patient as well as whether the variance can be resolved.

Many times, issues arise that were not known when the pathway was implemented, or the patient's condition may have changed since the pathway was started. A patient who is on a fractured hip pathway may develop variances when a comorbid condition, such as hypertension, complicates the treatment. In this case, the treatment would focus on treating the hypertension, since uncontrolled hypertension is life-threatening. The pathway for the treatment of the hip would be suspended until the hypertension was controlled, and a hypertension clinical pathway might be implemented. Once this is accomplished, the patient's care can return to the hip pathway. Often, care for both conditions, or any others, can proceed simultaneously.

Algorithms

Algorithms are systematic procedures that follow a logical progression according to additional information received or a patient's response to an intervention to reach a solution for a specific problem. Like protocols, algorithms are a series of treatment steps, each of which is defined by the clinical response of the patient to the preceding step. However, unlike protocols, algorithms are research-based and have scientific support data. One of the most recognized uses of algorithms is in advanced cardiac life support. Professionals use a specific algorithm that relates to specific cardiac rhythms. Corresponding treatment is designed to interrupt an abnormal rhythm in an attempt to normalize the rhythm. The use of algorithms helps to standardize emergency treatment, both inside the healthcare setting and in the community, to provide treatment in an organized and efficient manner and to achieve successful outcomes.

Decision Trees

Decision trees are used to select the best course of action in situations in which there are no clear decisions. Many businesses use decision trees to help them estimate how to determine inventories. An example is a manufacturing company that must decide how much inventory to build before knowing precisely what the demand will be. In the legal field, an example is a person who must choose between accepting an out-of-court settlement or risk the outcome of a trial. In health care, professionals must also make decisions without complete information. Decision-tree programs allow for the available information to be input into a program that systematically factors all variables so that a decision can be made. Many IT systems feature decision trees as part of standard software.

Case Simulation: Two nurses are working in the postop unit of a hospital. One nurse follows the clinical pathway developed for the care of patients who have had abdominal surgery; the other does not follow the established clinical pathway but documents her own care plan. The first nurse knows that pathways are care plans that detail the essential steps in the care of patients with a specific clinical problem and describe the expected progress of the patient; they exist for dozens of conditions or procedures. She performs each intervention at the prescribed time, as the patient tolerates. The second nurse, following her intuition instead of a pathway, tries to develop a care plan with her patient's input, which presents particular challenges when the patient is unconscious, semiconscious, woozy, or experiencing pain. The first nurse is able to begin her work with the patient even in his unconscious condition; she turns him, braces his abdomen with pillows, and checks all vital signs, medications, and so on. The second nurse is still assessing and documenting her care plan.

The result of this scenario was that the patient who was being cared for by the nurse following the unit's clinical pathway was transferred to a stepdown unit within the pathway's time line. The second patient being cared for by the second nurse creating her own care plan did not progress as well and was not ready to be transferred to the stepdown unit during this nurse's shift. This delayed transfer resulted in a backup in the OR schedule because of the lack of a postop bed. The end result was that the first patient's recovery was quicker, his transition between units smoother, and he was happier. This adherence to the clinical pathway also resulted in savings for the hospital.

Critical pathways or care maps are being implemented in a broad range of patients with many different diseases. Although cost savings can and should be evaluated with the critical pathway, improving guideline compliance and overall quality of care is the primary focus. Clinical protocols can and should be used to decrease variation in care, improve guideline compliance, and potentially improve overall quality of patient care. Practitioners and administrators should work together to incorporate clinical protocols and critical pathways, which may result in improved quality and reduced costs.

SCREENING TOOLS

The general concept of case management and care coordination is to educate people about how to improve their health status, to prevent or manage chronic illness, to improve quality of life, and to better control healthcare costs. To do this, healthcare professionals must understand how people view their own health status, comply with prescribed regimens, perform activities of daily living, and perceive quality of life. As a result, health plans and providers must seek valid methods of assessing health status of specific populations and respond to the need to identify at-risk members, to require clinical outcomes accountability, and to focus on population health management.

Health assessment screening tools can be useful in gathering this information. Health assessment screening tools allow providers to proactively evaluate a patient's perception of his or her health status, whether or not the patient understands the information given about a disease or injury, and the ongoing prognosis. After information has been given to a patient regarding a particular treatment or condition, a health assessment screening tool enables the practitioner to evaluate whether the patient understands and can apply the information, to maximize patient compliance. Should the screening tool show that the patient did not understand the information well enough to self-manage and achieve optimal results, referral to case management is indicated for reinforcement and monitoring of the patient's compliance and outcomes over time.

Health assessment screening tools are an effective means to evaluate risk and outcomes. However, they cannot be used to evaluate the implementation of interventions. The methods by which health assessment screening tools are implemented and used should be understood by the case manager, as well as by any member of the healthcare team using a health assessment screening tool.

Screening tools can be descriptive, predictive, or evaluative. A descriptive assessment tool collects data about the characteristics of a population to identify and implement health prevention in areas of greatest need.

Predictive tools are used to infer what may happen in a particular population, in particular disease conditions, or because of certain lifestyle behaviors. A predictive screening tool demonstrates factors among smokers, for example. Results show that smokers tend to develop more respiratory infections and chronic bronchitis than nonsmokers and recover from surgery more slowly.

Evaluative tools are survey tools that measure and weigh the effectiveness of a particular medical intervention or process. An example is a screening tool to measure outcomes of diabetic teaching to a population identified by a managed care organization using a disease management model (Ringel, 1998).

When developing screening tools, an interdisciplinary team that includes physicians is needed. The focus is on establishing and maintaining a streamlined process to make periodic health assessments a routine part of the care process, in both the inpatient and ambulatory settings. The most common screening tool used by providers and managed care organizations is the SF-36 Measurement Model.

The SF-36 is a multipurpose, short-form health survey with only 36 questions. It has been proven to be reliable and valid. It yields an eight-scale profile of functional health and well-being scores, as well as psychometrically based physical and mental health summary measures and a preference-based health utility index. It is a generic measure, as opposed to one that targets a specific age, disease, or treatment group. Accordingly, the SF-36 has proven useful in surveys of general and specific populations, comparing the relative burden of diseases, and in differentiating the health benefits produced by a wide range of different treatments.

The taxonomy has three levels: items, eight scales that aggregate between 2 and 10 items each, and two summary measures that aggregate scales. All but 1 of the 36 items (self-reported health transition) are used to score the eight SF-36 scales. Each item is used in scoring only one scale. The eight scales are hypothesized to form two distinct higher-ordered clusters because of the physical and mental health variance that they have in common (QualityMetric, 2012). The SF-12 measures general health status using the eight-scale profile, as seen in the SF-36. Results are expressed in two scores: the Physical Component Score and the Mental Component Summary (QualityMetric, 2012).

The Patient Activation Measure (PAM) is a 13-item tool that assesses patient knowledge, skill, and confidence for self-care. Scores range from 0 to 52, and a lower score indicates that the patient is less likely to have basic knowledge about his or her condition, treatment, or self-care. A PAM score can also predict healthcare outcomes, including medication adherence, ER use, and hospitalization (Insignia Health, 2012).

Health risk assessments (HRAs) can also be very effective in identifying patients who could benefit from aggressive outreach and interventions. HRAs evaluate a patient's perception of his or her current state of health. In addition, they are able to analyze results to determine whether or not the patient has an increased likelihood of seeking care. HRAs are able to predict not only future healthcare costs, but also the likelihood of progression toward illness or worsening of condition.

There are many such tools. Following is a list of some HRAs that case managers might find helpful in their daily work.

▶ **For angina:**

- Rose Questionnaire Seattle Angina Questionnaire

▶ **For arthritis:**

- Arthritis Impact Measurement Scales (AIMS)

▶ **For cancer:**

- Functional Living Index-Cancer

▶ **For mental status:**

- Basis-32
- Hopkins Symptom Checklist-25
- Mini-Mental State Examination

▶ **For pain:**

- McGill Pain Questionnaire
- MOS Pain Measures

▶ **For depression:**

- Patient Health Questionnaire 9
- Beck Depression Inventory

▶ **For attention-deficit hyperactivity disorder:**

- Vanderbilt Assessment Scale for Attention Deficit/Hyperactivity Disorder

▶ **For anxiety**

- Beck Anxiety Inventory

NURSING CASE MANAGEMENT PROCESSES

The case management process is an adapted version of the nursing process. Both are similar in that they identify a plan of care for patients by assessing needs, planning and implementing care, and evaluating outcomes. The difference is that the nursing process is applied to the care of every patient by all nurses in any care setting, whereas the case management process is used by case managers in the patient care delivery model and is applied only to a select group of patients who meet specific predetermined criteria.

TABLE 2-1.
COMPARISON OF THE NURSING PROCESS AND THE CASE MANAGEMENT PROCESS

CORE FUNCTIONS OF THE NURSING PROCESS	CORE FUNCTIONS OF THE CASE MANAGEMENT PROCESS
Assessment	Assessment
Diagnosis	n/a
Planning	Planning
Implementation	Implementation
n/a	Coordination and Interaction
Monitoring and Evaluation	Monitoring and Evaluation
n/a	Outcomes

Adapted from *The Case Manager's Survival Guide: Winning Strategies for Clinical Practice*, by T. G. Cesta, H. A. Tahan, and L. A. Fink, 2002, St. Louis, MO, Mosby.

Assessment

Assessment is the first essential function of the case management process. It is an organized, multidimensional progression by which the nurse case manager gathers and analyzes in-depth information in an attempt to understand the patient's physical, psychological, psychosocial, cognitive, functional, developmental, economic, cultural, spiritual, and lifestyle needs. To perform this task, the nurse case manager collects essential information from relevant sources, including the patient; his or her family; other healthcare professionals or institutions that have provided care; professional caregivers; employers; and public health, school, and military records. As a result of strict laws regarding confidentiality, nurse case managers should obtain a signed release from the patient and applicable family members prior to gathering the pertinent information.

An in-depth evaluation of the information provides valuable insight regarding the patient's history, as well as how the healthcare system has met his or her needs. Often, over- or underutilization of services becomes evident through this investigatory process. In addition, many patients use the healthcare system in inappropriate ways. As a result, services do not always match the true needs of the patient. It is the role of the nurse case manager to uncover any concerns about care.

Case Simulation: A patient with multiple chronic conditions has repeat admissions to the hospital. In order to understand the needs of the patient, the nurse case manager embarks on a comprehensive assessment that considers medical history, medications taken, previous hospitalizations, diagnostic tests and results, evaluations from specialists, and input from current providers, as well as the patient and his family. The information the nurse case manager collects during the assessment phase provides the team with the most up-to-date information before beginning an evaluation of the current condition, identifying unmet needs, clarifying and determining realistic goals, and deciding on a plan of care.

A complete and comprehensive assessment is critical to building a successful case management plan. Developing keen assessment skills is important if the nurse case manager is to make an accurate assessment of the patient's status and gain a better understanding of how the patient is dealing with his or her condition. Gathering this information allows the case manager to better assess the patient's needs and communicate these needs with the treatment team involved.

Physical and Clinical Issues of Assessment

The primary objective of the case management process is to ensure appropriate, high-quality care for at-risk individuals in a timely and cost-effective manner by providing services that are individualized, holistic, and meant to enhance self-care throughout the continuum. The tactics implemented to achieve the process objective include

▶ Helping the patient and his or her family achieve optimum function

▶ Coordinating the delivery of care

▶ Decreasing fragmentation and ensuring appropriate use of resources

▶ Enhancing the quality of life for the individual patient and his or her family

▶ Improving and facilitating interdisciplinary communication and planning

▶ Helping to strengthen the family unit when injury and illness strike through support, empowerment, and effective and efficient care coordination

▶ Maximizing the health of patients by increasing healthcare education that promotes wellness

▶ Proactively identifying problems and needs, and implementing services that provide appropriate, high-quality care to meet the individualized needs of the patient and his or her family.

Nurse case managers work in various settings throughout the continuum of care. Traditionally, organizations that have implemented case management systems have created their own models that correlate to the organizations' operations. In addition, these organizations can target case management to specific patient populations, communities, or departments. Examples include children, the elderly, and those with mental illness, or specific areas, such as the emergency department, to assist patients with appropriate access to the healthcare system.

Psychosocial Issues of Assessment

Another aspect of the nurse case manager's assessment focuses on psychosocial issues that impact a patient's life. Some questions a case manager can ask to gain insight include:

▶ What are the family dynamics?

▶ Is the patient a child, mother, or father, or is the patient single or a widow or widower?

▶ What is the patient's educational level?

▶ Is the patient a citizen of the United States?

▶ If no, when did he or she arrive in the United States?

▶ What is the patient's primary spoken language?

▶ Is the patient an active member of his or her community?

▶ Does the patient feel that he or she has a social network in place?

▶ Does the patient work, or is he or she retired or disabled?

▶ Does the patient have any hobbies?

▶ What is his or her spiritual affiliation?

The answers to these and other similar questions shed light on the life of the patient and allow the nurse case manager to assess whether the patient will need assistance with providing self-care or has the necessary support to fight the challenges of a catastrophic or chronic condition. In addition, the answers also provide insight into any possible literacy issues that might hinder patient education. The answers provide important clues for better understanding the patient and family dynamics, and should play a part in the patient assessment.

Case Simulation: Two patients in the midst of a similar healthcare crisis reveal very different social, economic, and financial dynamics and, therefore, very different needs. Patient one is a father of two. He has a supportive family, has been working for the same employer for 15 years, and is an active member of his community and church. Patient number two is a divorced mother of three children. She works two jobs just to get by, has no local family to speak of, and relies on neighbors for after-school care. The assessment reveals that she has significantly more needs and requires more support.

Developmental Issues of Assessment

Nurse case managers need to understand growth and development patterns of their patients. This is especially true for the nurse case manager who specializes in pediatrics. Understanding normal growth and development patterns is necessary to ensure that the care provided is illness- and age-specific. To understand the developmental patterns of children and better prepare to address issues that may arise when children experience health challenges, case managers should take time to review the work of three pediatric theorists. These theorists provide insight into the stages of growth and development by age group.

▶ Jean Piaget (1896–1980) was a cognitive theorist who addressed children's abilities by age group to synthesize and analyze information. Piaget's theory can help the nurse case manager understand why reasoning with young children about the need for a procedure is not possible. Instead, encouraging parents and caregivers to support and comfort children during and after procedures may prove more effective.

Case Simulation: When educating the mother of a 5-year-old with cystic fibrosis about performing chest percussions, the case manager would not tell the mother to give the child a choice of when to do the therapy. Instead, comforting the child and spending time doing something he or she likes after therapy is a better way to approach the child's expected resistance.

▶ Erik Erickson (1902–1994) focused on children's social environments. His work helps case managers to understand peer pressure felt by children, which may make them noncompliant with medication or treatment regimes.

Case Simulation: An adolescent who is newly diagnosed with diabetes is having high blood sugars and admits to hating the foods she has to eat because of her diabetes. The nurse case manager realizes that teenagers want to "fit in," so following a diabetic diet is a challenge. Understanding and acknowledging peer pressure, the nurse case manager consults with a nutritionist to provide a diet that allows some flexibility when the teenager is out with friends. By doing this, the case manager provides a way for the teen to "fit in" without compromising her health.

▶ B. F. Skinner (1904–1990) focused on behavior. His research with monkeys proved the effectiveness of a reward system for appropriate behavior. Bargaining is an effective tool that works when dealing with school-age children who are rewarded with special favors or favorite television shows when they comply with treatments.

Case Simulation: A child with a chronic illness might feel less important than his peers. Rewarding him for taking his medication or doing his exercises daily is a way to boost his self-esteem, while at the same time helping him learn how to manage his illness.

Financial Issues of Assessment

The United States spends more on health per capita than any other country. Projected healthcare spending for 2012 in the United States will reach $3.1 trillion, or 17.1% of the gross national product (Henry J. Kaiser Family Foundation, 2012). For case management to successfully help control escalating healthcare costs, early identification of at-risk populations is essential. In cases of sudden catastrophic illness or injury, early referral to case management services is important to ensure that the patient is admitted to the appropriate facility and moves through the system in a coordinated manner that will meet his or her medical needs. For those who suffer from chronic illness or progressive disease, the need for case management services is determined by how the patient and the family are handling their specific challenges. Screening tools provide the healthcare team with information about the patient's perception of his or her illness. This information helps with early identification of those patients who need help improving their health status, thus avoiding or minimizing potentially costly problems.

Case Simulation: A patient with diabetes who is seen in the emergency department (ED) several times for problems related to dizziness and blurred vision is referred to the ED case manager on his most recent visit. The case manager takes the time to talk to the patient about the reasons for his frequent visits, to review lab results, and to discuss the clinical picture with both the ED physician and the patient—all in an effort to gain a better understanding of how the patient is managing his illness. The nurse case manager learns that the patient does not have a primary care physician because he has no health insurance because he lost his job. As a result of taking the time to talk with the patient, the case manager can assist him with access to appropriate resources that will result in decreased fragmentation of care, improved quality of care, and reduced costs associated with misuse of resources.

As part of the process of assessment, the nurse case manager reviews available benefits, including those for services and products, for the patient and his family. This requires the case manager to have a working knowledge of various reimbursement systems. Plans can vary from commercial managed care plans, such as health maintenance organization (HMO) and preferred provider organization (PPO) plans, to traditional indemnity plans in which there is no network of providers and much greater financial risk. Likewise, patients may have Medicare with special rider policies to supplement their coverage. Since Medicaid plans vary from state to state, the hospital case manager might negotiate discharge planning for two Medicaid patients with vastly different postacute benefits and available resources. Patients also may enter the healthcare system through the workers' compensation system, which requires constant communication with the primary care physician, nurse case manager, claims adjustor, and employer. Taking the time to become familiar with the various reimbursement systems is important because each has very specific reimbursement guidelines. These are covered in greater detail in Chapter 3.

Planning

The next essential function for the nursing case management process is planning. Planning is the process by which the nurse case manager develops a patient-centered, evidence-based, interdisciplinary plan of care based upon complete analysis of data. The nurse case manager collaborates with the patient, family, caregivers, healthcare team, payer, and other stakeholders, as needed, to develop an individualized plan of care. This comprehensive plan is focused, action-oriented, time-specific, evidence-based, measurable, attainable, fiscally responsible, and interdisciplinary. The nurse case management plan contains short- and long-term, patient-centered goals that are reviewed and updated as the patient moves through the continuum of care. Its goal is to provide high-quality care that meets the needs of the patient in the most cost-effective manner. The plan prioritizes the needs of the patient and strives to meet those immediate needs, while moving the patient through the continuum of care in the least restrictive settings.

Depending on the timelines of the case management plan, it can start in one setting and continue in another. Ideally, the same nurse case manager follows the patient from one setting to the next. However, in reality, moving to each level of care may result in a new case manager.

Case Simulation: A patient making the transition from the acute care setting to a rehabilitation facility and then back home with the support of home health care has four case managers coordinating her care—the acute care nurse case manager, the rehabilitation case manager, the home health case manager, and the payer case manager. The case manager responsible for transferring the patient from one setting to the next ensures that detailed information is provided regarding what was done, what the future plan is, and why the transfer is taking place. Documentation presenting the rationale for the transfer is important to ensure a safe and effective transition of care.

A key question that the nurse case manager should ask and be able to answer is: "What is the clinical evidence that allows this patient to move safely from one setting to the other?" The answer to this question provides the rationale for the transfer. Specific rules apply to the transfer of patients from one setting to another, so it is important that all case managers be aware of the policies and follow them to guard against inappropriate transfers.

The case manager works collaboratively with the treatment team to develop the plan of care and then obtains approval for the plan from the treating physician, the patient, the family, and the payer. Depending on the payer source, the case manager may need to obtain authorization for the plan of care prior to implementation, a step that should be considered at the planning phase. Authorization is especially important in the area of workers' compensation, as well as with some commercial managed care organizations. It is important that the nurse case manager be aware of the cost of the plan that is being constructed to ensure that it cost-effectively meets that patient's needs. If funding is not available but the services are needed, the nurse case manager works to gain approval or negotiates with the payer to see how to utilize the benefits to meet the needs of the patient.

The nurse case manager must recognize that denial of payment for services from the payer is not the final word. As an advocate for the patient, the case manager must look at what is medically necessary and strive to find resources to safely ensure that those services are provided. This may mean asking for an exception to the benefit plan, utilizing community resources, or extending the patient's stay in the current setting. A safe and appropriate discharge is essential to any case management plan.

Finally, it is important that the plan of care be documented; it is a dynamic document that is referred to on an ongoing basis.

Implementation

Implementation is the third essential function in the case management process. It is the execution of the specific case management activities and interventions that lead to accomplishing the goals set forth in the plan of care. Implementation includes proactive activities such as intervening, delegating, facilitating, goal-setting, and communicating. Once the plan is developed and approved by the treating physician, the payer, and the patient and family, it is implemented by the nurse case manager. Using negotiation skills, the nurse case manager works to ensure that services begin in a coordinated manner among the various providers, the patient, and the family. Through careful planning, knowledge of resources, and appropriate communication, duplication of services is avoided and fragmentation is reduced. The end result: the patient receives care that is appropriate, timely, and cost-effective.

The ability of the nurse case manager to implement and coordinate a successful plan of care is influenced by his or her level of education, training, and clinical expertise. For example, an advanced practice nurse has the specialized skills, knowledge, and ability to effect change, use critical thinking, promote patient and family autonomy, build positive relationships, and understand and interpret research for enhanced decision-making. Using these skill sets when implementing challenging plans of care is essential to successful outcomes.

Goal-Setting

It is important for the nurse case manager to formulate goals in concert with the patient, family, and caregiver. Setting goals gives the plan of care structure and a means to measure and report outcomes in an organized manner. Goals should be patient-focused, measurable, attainable, relevant, and time-orientated. The patient, as well as the family, should take part in the development of short- and long-term goals. By working closely with the patient and his or her family, the case manager gains an understanding of the needs of the patient, the diagnosis, and the treatment plan, as well as insight into the patient's lifestyle, personal habits, attitudes, and well-being.

An important goal the nurse case manager strives to achieve is adherence to the plan of care. Adherence is pivotal to achieving desired heath outcomes. The effectiveness of the case management process is based upon the linkages between interventions, adherence, and outcomes.

Negotiating

Effective case managers are skillful negotiators. The basic skill for a successful negotiation is the ability to build solid relationships among all parties involved. The level of trust, knowledge, and flexibility of those involved in the negotiation process influences the success of any negotiation. When the nurse case manager takes the time to understand what motivates the individual members of the patient care team, which includes the patient and his or her family, negotiations are more likely to succeed.

Managed care has decreased the need for price negotiations because of provider contracts that are set up in advance. Today, the nurse case manager is viewed as the negotiator of care rather than the negotiator of costs. This broader view allows the case manager to consider the entire process, rather than focus solely on costs. As part of the plan development, the nurse case manager is obligated to ensure that the services and products put into place are medically necessary, priced appropriately, and delivered with high-quality service.

Case Simulation: A transplant patient requires costly medication for life. The nurse case manager negotiated with three network vendors for the lowest possible price. The savings generated by the negotiated lower rate is reported as cost savings. These cost savings allow for the more effective use of benefit dollars, thereby meeting the patient's needs over a longer period of time.

Contracting

For managed care to effectively manage risk within an organization's network, providers and vendors who can adequately provide services to meet the healthcare needs of the members are selected. Several factors are taken into consideration when a managed care plan develops its provider network, such as the demographic and geographic makeup of its members. Providers seeking to join a managed care organization's network must meet certain criteria and standards. Standards are set by the managed care network, by a state legislative agency if the state mandates that managed care networks exist, or by an accreditation organization. These requirements are necessary to ensure that the providers in the network follow the standards set by the managed care organization and by imposed legislation. Policies and procedures are usually reviewed on an annual basis when provider contracts are renewed. Once a contract is signed and the provider is credentialed, the provider can begin to serve members in the managed care organization.

For example, acute care hospitals, home care agencies, and durable medical equipment (DME) companies might require accreditation by The Joint Commission before ever being considered as a network provider. During the credentialing phase, the provider must supply documentation of review by The Joint Commission. This information is important because the managed care organization is responsible for selecting providers who can offer high-quality care for their members.

Finally, providers who join a managed care network must agree to the reimbursement rate—usually based on capitation—that the organization offers. The provider is paid a fixed fee, which cannot be altered despite how often the provider's services are accessed.

Coordination and Interaction

Coordination and interaction are essential and inherent to all phases of the case management process. These components consist of organizing, securing, integrating, and modifying the resources necessary to accomplish the goals set forth in the case management plan. As part of this process, the nurse case manager must be aware of the cost of both current and recommended care in order to ensure that suggested interventions are cost-effective. When possible, community resources are used. The nurse case manager is cognizant of and compliant with regulations, standards, and legislation at the local, state, and national levels. Essential competency skills for the nurse case manager who coordinates an individualized plan of care are effective communication, collaboration, assertiveness, and cooperation with all parties.

As mentioned earlier, coordinating a safe and effective plan of care is critical to the success of the plan. The case manager must verify that the patient and the family understand the plan of care and that the various contracted providers understand their roles in the process. The nurse case manager validates that interventions are consistent with the established plan of care and that the plan is implemented in a safe and timely manner. The case manager who initiates the plan, if not following the case through the continuum of care, should make a follow-up call to be certain that all aspects of the plan are in place. By proactively addressing problems regarding the plan, the case manager can intervene early to make changes as needed. If problems are found, the case manager assesses the situation and develops measures to address it.

In many cases, once the patient leaves a specific setting, such as the hospital, interaction with the nurse case manager ends. In other cases, however, a new case manager may take over. It's important to understand that a smooth transition is possible when communication and collaboration occur among all parties. The patient and the family should receive instructions about how to follow up if they have questions or concerns about any aspect of the plan of care. Documentation of all case management activities is the final detail in this process.

Collaboration

Collaboration is an essential skill that the nurse case manager uses to unite the members of the healthcare team and others who are integral to designing a plan of care for an individual patient. Collaboration by the case manager fosters consistency, which reduces fragmentation and duplication of services. Effective collaboration ensures patient and provider satisfaction, an important outcome that all healthcare organizations strive to achieve. The timely delivery and sensitive handling of information by the nurse case manager are essential to ensuring patient confidentiality and relevant decision-making. When pertinent information is communicated to providers in a timely manner, the nurse case manager ensures that decisions are made with full information, thus decreasing duplication of services.

Consultation and Referrals

Consultation is the act of conferring with another individual in order to gain an opinion or advice. One person usually consults with another because the second person is considered an expert who can give professional advice or services. Consultation is a large part of the fact-finding and assessment stage in case management. However, consultation with other members of the healthcare team continues throughout all phases of the case management process and is one of the defining factors to create a holistic, objective, and effective plan of care.

Once the referral process is completed, the nurse case manager employs his or her clinical skills in a comprehensive, fact-finding assessment process. It is the nurse case manager's responsibility to conduct a thorough and objective evaluation of the patient's current status, including medical, financial, psychological, social, and vocational aspects. To accomplish this, the nurse case manager needs to collaborate with the family, physicians, and other members of the healthcare team, as well as the payer and employer (if any). Understanding the unique aspects of each member of the team is important.

Case management has improved the delivery of health care by encouraging the team to work together instead of in silos. The following three examples illustrate how members of the healthcare team collaborate to meet the needs of the patient.

▶ **The physician:** The key decision-maker regarding the patient's treatment plan, and often the most important consultant to the clinical case manager, is the physician. Although the physician is responsible for diagnosing and treating the patient, he or she relies on the input and suggestions from the case manager and other members of the healthcare team on how to best meet the patient's needs. The nurse case manager, who has a unique relationship with the patient and the family, provides valuable insight that can assist all in developing an effective and efficient plan of care.

A nurse case manager who has developed a positive relationship with a physician is in an advantageous position to facilitate the patient's case management care plan by

  ▸ Suggesting potential alternatives to the treatment plan that can enhance quality of care while lowering costs;

  ▸ Arranging out-of-benefit resources covered by the payer based on a letter of medical necessity from the physician and supporting documentation;

  ▸ Initiating a discussion between the payer's medical director and the patient's physician, which can result in better care for the patient;

  ▸ Enlisting the physician in problem-solving on a current or future difficult case; or

  ▸ Using the physician as an informational resource or an actual referral source for other cases.

▶ **The pharmacist:** Another key member of the healthcare team is the pharmacist. The increased role that pharmacy and drug management play in healthcare delivery makes it essential for the nurse case manager to consult regularly with pharmacists. Biological and technological advances in medicine continue to escalate the use of high-cost medications in the treatment of complicated conditions. With this comes an increase in the incidence of drug interactions, drug sensitivity, drug overdose, and polypharmacy. Polypharmacy is a critical issue among many patients with complex chronic conditions, and pharmacists are in a key position to curb or eliminate this potentially dangerous situation.

Pharmacists can assist the case manager in understanding the various prescribing habits of physicians or help strategize an approach with the patient's physician when attempting to suggest a potential alternative drug intervention. Pharmacists are excellent resources for those cases in which the patient is prescribed a battery of drugs, and the nurse case manager is engaged in educating the patient, which requires knowledge of drugs' indications, side effects, and so forth. Pharmacists are great allies for the case manager dealing with a noncompliant or nonadherent patient. They can assist in monitoring the patient's medication compliance, as well as offer education and support resources to the patient to increase compliance. Pharmacists are also an excellent source of information for the patient and a vital link in establishing a relationship with the patient that is built upon trust.

▶ **The clinical nurse:** As highly skilled clinicians, nurses are excellent consultants and good sources of information for the case manager. Staff nurses are reliable historians when dealing with a patient in an acute care setting, rehabilitation facility, or long-term-care facility. They

  ▹ Report on a patient's physical, mental, and behavioral status;

  ▹ Provide insight into family dynamics;

  ▹ Assess the patient's ongoing responsiveness to the treatment plan; and

  ▹ Are trained to view the patient holistically, much as the nurse case manager is, making them a valuable resource to the clinical case manager.

Often, bedside nurses care for a particular patient because of their expertise in that patient's specific disease or injury. Therefore, they are also excellent sources of information pertaining to the patient's diagnosis and prognosis.

Collaboration among all members of the healthcare team occurs in a variety of ways and through a variety of venues—by ongoing one-on-one telephone communication or shared teleconference calls, by providing written narrative reports to all parties, by sharing charting and documentation that is e-mailed for review and group comment, and through face-to-face meetings. Confidentiality issues regarding the patient's right to privacy arise with each of these communication methods, and the nurse case manager must be aware of policies and procedures that address who, what, when, and how a patient's medical information is shared.

Acute care case managers have the greatest advantage in collaborating with the interdisciplinary team, especially when they engage in regularly scheduled team staffing meeting or rounds. Clinical rounds and staff meetings engage all members of the healthcare team and allow sharing of information about the patient's response to treatment.

Communication Skills

Interpersonal communication: Verbal and written communication skills are essential for nurse case managers. As the professional at the center of the team, the nurse case manager must interpret complex, detailed clinical and financial information, and disseminate that information—both orally and in written form—to others who need to know. To be successful, the nurse case manager takes a vast amount of information and summarizes it, without distortion or imposing personal judgment. When talking to other healthcare professionals, the case manager must be prepared with concise questions that help providers understand what is being asked and, therefore, provide information to that explains or clarifies the patient's condition.

A popular expression that nurse case managers should keep in mind is: *your emergency is not my emergency*. With this in mind, the nurse case manager must respect the time of others when requesting information. In addition to demands on other people's time, the nurse case manager, who talks with a variety of people, ranging from highly educated professionals to laypersons, should consider the educational level of the person with whom he or she is communicating. Effective communication with ethnically diverse populations may require the use of interpreter or translation services. Another essential communication skill is the ability to listen. The case manager learns a great deal by listening and observing those with whom he or she interacts.

Information is also obtained and transmitted in written form. Often, the nurse case manager composes letters to be mailed, faxed, or sent via e-mail to treating physicians or providers, requesting information to help clarify or update the plan of care, or offering details of a revised treatment plan. The effective nurse case manager must be aware of patient privacy legislation and how it applies to all forms of communication and needs to comply appropriately.

Accurate documentation is an essential form of communication to describe outcomes and improve the process of case management. Written documentation is viewed as the permanent record that specifies, summarizes, analyzes, and synthesizes verbal and nonverbal data that support the work and time that a nurse case manager gives to each patient.

Critical thinking and problem-solving: As nurse case managers increase their presence in the healthcare system, the need for critical thinking and the ability to problem-solve become more crucial. To achieve effective outcomes in today's healthcare environment, the nurse case manager must have skills that ensure problem identification in a proactive manner, and timely resolution. An organized approach uses the following strategies to ensure effective problem-solving:

- ▶ Identify the issue
- ▶ Understand each party's issue
- ▶ List possible solutions
- ▶ Evaluate the outcomes
- ▶ Select an option or options
- ▶ Agree on contingencies, monitoring, and evaluation (Hicks, 2007).

The traits needed by nurse case managers to critically think and problem-solve include excellent communication skills, organizational skills, flexibility, and creativity. By using critical thinking skills, the case manager is able to identify problems, investigate solutions, and work to ensure that a timely resolution occurs to maintain continuity of care.

As healthcare professionals, nurse case managers are required to interact with patients and families during very personal and stressful times. Astute case managers have the opportunity to use their expertise to recognize potential conflicts and put measures in place that address and resolve conflicts in a way that is agreeable to all. To resolve conflicts, the nurse case manager must be able to encourage and maintain open communication and facilitate a positive flow of ideas among all parties with whom interactions occur.

Case Simulation: A workers' compensation nurse case manager's main goal is to assist an injured worker in returning to gainful employment. In accomplishing this goal, the case manager interacts with the employer, the injured worker, and the treating physician. On a visit with the patient to the treating physician, the case manager learns that the injured worker, who is a tree trimmer, is able to return to work but with restrictions of only working 4 hours a day. The case manager calls the employer to update him regarding the treating physician's plan of care, but the employer says that he cannot use someone who can only work 4 hours because this would put hardship on the rest of the staff. To resolve this conflict, the nurse case manager explains to the employer the benefits that he will derive from bringing the employee back to work. The employer remembers he has a drawer filled with addresses of potential clients that he has not had time to contact. The case manager works with the employer and helps him formulate a plan to bring the injured worker back to work to build a database of potential clients. The nurse case manager takes this opportunity to explain to the employer that bringing this employee back to work may keep the company's future workers' compensation rates from increasing. Also, morale will be improved when other workers see that the employer is willing to accommodate an employee who was injured. Finally, the nurse case manager reminds the employer that the injured worker, who is being paid whether he works or not, will be more productive to the employer by being at work. The case manager discusses the duties with the injured worker, and he happily returns to work; he was tired of sitting at home and glad that his employer found something he could do while he continued to heal.

In this situation, the case manager showed a positive outcome by using negotiating skills to offset a potential conflict. It was a win for the employer, who was able to have someone who could assist him in the development of a database of potential clients that would hopefully expand his business, and a win for the injured worker, who was able to return to work within his restrictions. The case manager stayed involved to assist with any problems and to communicate the patient's progress to the treating physicians. The case manager documented the information in the injured worker's file, showing that the injured worker returned to work following the physician's instructions and that the employer safely accommodated him in the work setting. The nurse case manager showed a successful outcome and reported cost savings on the claim with an early return to work and a decrease in lost time.

Monitoring and Evaluation

The final essential concepts in the case management process, aside from outcomes, are monitoring and evaluation. To ensure that the plan of care is meeting the established goals, the nurse case manager monitors the plan of care on a continuing basis by gathering information from the providers involved to show that the plan implemented is effectively meeting goals. Proactive monitoring of the plan ensures that the patient is making progress toward the desired outcomes. If progress is not being made, modifications or changes to the plan in its entirety, or in specific components, are made as needed.

Evaluation provides the nurse case manager an opportunity to improve the plan of care if it is not meeting the goals or if the patient is not making progress. The evaluation is part of the continuous quality improvement process that organizations and accreditation bodies require. In addition, the evaluation process gives the nurse case manager time to review providers to ensure that all contracted services are consistent with the organization's standards. The evaluation process gives the case manager the opportunity to review the achievement of specific goals outlined in the plan of care and the chance to demonstrate the importance of his or her role in the case.

Outcomes Measurement

Once an individualized plan of care is crafted, the nurse case manager is responsible for initiating the interventions and monitoring the plan's effectiveness. Specifying goals at the onset of care planning allows the nurse case manager to evaluate the effectiveness of those goals as a result of the nurse case manager's involvement.

From a global view, evaluation of outcomes is an integral part of the quality improvement process. All information about outcomes—successful or not—should be reported. This information allows providers and practitioners to focus on systems' structures and to make changes as needed to improve both systems and individualized practice.

With the development and implementation of information systems, decision-makers can analyze large amounts of data. This allows them to choose a course of action that has the highest expectation of favorable results, in terms of both clinical and financial impacts. Through careful evaluation of the data, changes, procedures, and policies can be reviewed and adjusted as needed, thereby improving systems.

Patient Adherence to Plan of Care

Adherence to a plan of care implies a relationship in which the patient and his or her healthcare providers come to a consensus on the most appropriate treatment that he or she can and will follow. The World Health Organization defines adherence as:

> the extent to which a person's behavior—taking medications, following a diet and/or executing lifestyle changes—corresponds with agreed recommendations from a health care provider. The consequence of nonadherence to the plan of care can result in a decrease in quality of life as well as unnecessary increases in avoidable health care cost. (Sabate, 2003, p. 3)

An important goal among nurse case managers is to work with their patients toward adherence to the prescribed plan of care. A case manager tackles this by taking the time to listen to the patient and to understand the goals and barriers that lead to nonadherence. Often, obstacles to adherence can be overcome. Once these problems are identified, the case manager can work with the patient to remove the barriers. Taking the time to educate the patient regarding the purpose of the treatment and the intended outcomes is important, as is learning what motivates the patient to better adhere to the treatment.

Services

Case managers receive referrals from various sources. These include integrated delivery systems, insurance company in-house triage systems, outside insurance adjusters, third-party administrators, acute and postacute healthcare facilities, social service agencies, attorneys, employers, federal systems, other healthcare professionals, and patients and their families. Because of this, how case managers initiate interventions varies greatly.

The way in which a nurse case manager approaches a new case is greatly influenced by the referral source and the payer system. Issues such as insurance policy limits, available coverage, eligibility for benefits, available funds, and other fiscal issues are considered when determining a plan of care. Yet it is the case manager's responsibility to exercise fiscal responsibility when accepting a referral, receiving a patient into a facility, or arranging a discharge.

Case Simulation: An acute care facility has a clear financial advantage in keeping a patient. However, the case manager knows that the patient could receive high-quality care with a less intensive level of service, such as a subacute facility or even in the patient's home. The case manager, aware of her responsibility, recommends discharge to the appropriate service location, regardless of financial incentives. Another patient who has exceeded the benefits under his health plan continues to require services in a healthcare facility. Rather than close the case, the case manager explores and identifies appropriate community services, and arranges the patient's transfer once a new plan is implemented.

Pathophysiology

To help individuals better cope with chronic illness, nurse case managers must understand the pathophysiological and psychological aspects of the disease process so that they can encourage patients and families to make positive behavioral changes and learn self-management skills that will allow them to more readily adapt to their conditions. When patients are empowered to self-manage, adherence to the plan of care increases, techniques are used to better manage complications, and disability is minimized.

Once an individual is identified as having been diagnosed with a chronic illness, a multidisciplinary team of experts constructs a proactive program to address the diverse needs of the patient. These experts work closely with the patient's physician or nurse practitioner because he or she is legally licensed to diagnose and treat the patient and, therefore, is the most appropriate provider to determine the treatment plan.

Case Simulation: A respiratory therapist case manager monitors and educates an asthma patient, who started on a new routine of using a peak flow meter. She explains that the meter, which measures lung capacity and functional levels, can help the patient better manage activities and self-adjust medications to fit his physical and functional requirements. She shows the patient how to accurately read the meter and be cognizant of alerts to conditions that require immediate medical attention, such as an upper respiratory infection that can trigger an acute episode of wheezing. Early identification of asthma triggers allows the patient to adjust medications to control attacks. By developing a routine of regularly measuring peak flows, the patient has learned to recognize whether preventive measures are working or if he needs to seek medical attention.

The outcomes that this particular asthma disease management program can claim just through this singular proactive education are

- ► Improved patient and provider satisfaction,
- ► Improved clinical status,
- ► Improved functional status,
- ► Appropriate use of healthcare resources,
- ► Decreases in lost time at work or school, and
- ► Decreases in healthcare spending on reactive care.

Psychosocial Conditions

Chronic diseases take patients and families through periods of good health mixed v [...] of sickness. During these times, patients experience a variety of emotions that can o [...] complicate care. To support and empower patients and families to develop coping strategies, case managers are aware that each person reacts and handles problems in his or her own way. Listening to patients and family members about how they are coping is a vital skill for case managers. Understanding the impact a chronic illness or catastrophic injury has on family dynamics is also important.

Relaying this information to other members of the healthcare team in an effort to help them understand the challenges and stressors that affect the patient is an important function of the nurse case manager. Being sensitive to the range of emotions that patients experience (e.g., denial, confusion, fear, avoidance, anger, grief, guilt) allows the nurse case manager to better understand why the patient and family act in a particular way (National Institutes of Health, 1996).

Providing support to the patient and family during these times is essential. This may entail referral to social services, guidance on how to sign up for community support groups, or recommendations for online support programs. The objective is that the patient and his and her family become aware of the various options available to them.

CMAG and IM-CAG

Two tools that are useful for pathophysiologial and psychological assessment are the Case Management Adherence Guidelines (CMAG) and the INTERMED-Complexity Assessment Grid (IM-CAG). CMAG is a comprehensive model based on patient information, motivation, and behavior skill needs. It provides a comprehensive approach to addressing issues relating to chronic therapies (CMSA, 2006–2007). These guidelines are available for medication adherence and disease-specific guidelines on cardiometabolic risk, chronic obstructive pulmonary disease, deep venous thrombosis, and diabetes.

IM-CAG is a valid, electronic tool designed to provide a picture of risks and vulnerabilities of complex patients with actionable interventions. A core component of the IM-CAG training program is the ability to assist patients with complexity and aid them in receiving integrated physical and mental health services without cross-disciplinary "hand-offs." Failure to treat depression can prevent proper treatment of other medical conditions because the depressed patient lacks the motivation or desire to improve his or her health (Karthal, Perez, Cohen, 2010). IM-CAG has four domains—behavioral, social, biological, and health system—with three time frames: historical, current, and anticipated. Scoring is based on the patient's vulnerability and need for action. More information on CMAG and IM-CAG can be found at www.cmsa.org.

Evidence-Based Practice

Evidence-based practice (EBP) is a thoughtful integration of the best available evidence, coupled with clinical expertise. As such, it enables health practitioners of all disciplines to address healthcare questions with an evaluative and qualitative approach. EBP allows the practitioner to assess current and past research, clinical guidelines, and other information resources in order to identify relevant literature while differentiating between high- and low-quality findings. The practice of EBP includes five fundamental steps:

Step 1: Formulating a well-built question

Step 2: Identifying articles and other evidence-based resources that answer the question

Step 3: Critically appraising the evidence to assess its validity

Step 4: Applying the evidence

Step 5: Reevaluating the application of evidence and areas for improvement (Schmidt & Brown, 2008)

Why Evidence-Based Practice?

From a policy perspective: In 1997, the Agency for Health Care Policy and Research (AHCPR), now known as the Agency for Healthcare Research and Quality (AHRQ), launched its initiative to promote evidence-based practice in everyday care through establishment of 14 Evidence-based Practice Centers (EPCs). The EPCs develop evidence reports and technology assessments on topics relevant to clinical, social science and behavioral, economic, and other healthcare organization and delivery issues—specifically those that are common, expensive, significant, or a combination of these for the Medicare and Medicaid populations. With this program, AHRQ became a "science partner" with private and public organizations in their efforts to improve the quality, effectiveness, and appropriateness of health care by synthesizing the evidence and facilitating the translation of evidence-based research findings. Topics are nominated by nonfederal partners such as professional societies, health plans, insurers, employers, and patient groups (AHRQ, 2011).

Three factors have influenced the development of EBP:

► An explosion of literature: For example, there are more than 7,800 articles relevant to family practice published monthly (Alper, Hand, et al., 2004).

► Unmet information needs among practitioners: For every three patients seen, two questions are generated. Because of a lack of time, lack of information resources, and poor researching skills, only 30% of these questions get answered during the patient's visit (Covell, Uman, & Manning, 1985).

► Slow or delayed implementation: Research findings are often delayed in being implemented into clinical practice. It takes an average of 17 years for clinical research to be fully integrated into everyday practice (Balas & Boren, 2000). Consider back- versus stomach-sleeping for infants. Prior to the early 1990s, it was recommended that infants sleep on their stomachs despite evidence available in the 1970s that stomach-sleeping contributed to sudden infant death syndrome (Gilbert, Salanti, & Harden, & See, 2005).

Therefore, it is clear why evidence-based practice has become a significant process for managing quality. The idea of EBP for nursing has grown out of the evidence-based medicine movement. Nurse case managers can use it to integrate their individual clinical expertise with the best available external clinical evidence from research. At its best, evidence-based practice gives the case manager the necessary tools to help enhance clinical effectiveness and affect the delivery of health care based on the integration of research, clinical guidelines, and outcomes' assessments into clinical practice.

Case Simulation: A 52-year-old man with a history of knee pain from osteoarthritis of the joint visits his provider's office and mentions that a coworker has suggested electrical nerve stimulation— also known as TENS (transcutaneous electrical nerve stimulation)—to relieve his symptoms. The provider needs to find some solid evidence that TENS has been used successfully to relieve knee pain. The provider must first formulate a well-built question: What effect, if any, does TENS have on chronic knee pain? The provider must then identify articles and other evidence-based resources that answer the question. The provider also needs to critically appraise the evidence to assess its validity. Did it come from a credible source? Did the studies conducted show significant, valid evidence? Next the provider applies the evidence. If he found that his patient met criteria similar to that for patients in the studies' target populations, he could write a prescription for the service. After the recommended period of time for application of TENS, he would reevaluate the patient to determine the effectiveness of the treatment.

Many different resources can help case managers research evidence-based health care. Textbooks, handbooks, databases, and articles are available online. Two popular Web sites are Ovid CINAHL (www.ebscohost.com/cinahl) and MEDLINE (www.MEDLINE.com). Case managers also need to know how to critically look at research articles to determine their validity and appropriateness. The American Academy of Family Physicians (AAFP; www.aafp.org/online/en/home.html) is a useful resource for finding critical appraisals of research articles. Journals that publish critiques of original research articles can help case managers judge the quality of original research, too. Examples of these journals include the ACP Journal Club Collection and BMJ Guidelines (www.bmj.com). Both journals look for original research and systematic reviews that may be of widespread importance to clinicians. Each presents a brief review of the research or systematic review.

Without EBP, case managers may see inadequate care, significant variations in practice, an increase in healthcare costs, and an increase in morbidity and mortality. It is imperative that case managers employ best practices for high-quality outcomes and cost-effective care.

Integrated Case Management

Today's health care is fragmented. Thus, one of the greatest challenges for patients with chronic medical conditions and concurrent mental health needs, often those with the highest health service use, is to receive coordinated care and assistance that will stabilize medical and mental health symptoms while also addressing social and health system factors that contribute to poor outcomes. This is aggravated by the fact that case managers with medical backgrounds do not feel competent to assist with mental health needs, and those with mental health backgrounds do not feel competent to deal with medical needs (CMSA, 2010). Integrated case management (ICM) is a comprehensive, advanced care management program that incorporates all medical management functions—utilization management, case management, disease management, triage, and prevention and wellness—to manage and deploy resources to optimize clinical, quality, and financial outcomes. ICM goes beyond traditional case and disease management in that it:

▶ Is proactive, collaborative, and patient-centric

▶ Is multidisciplinary across all settings

▶ Focuses on improved health status and quality of care

▶ Streamlines processes and improves resource management

▶ Enhances communication and documentation

▶ Coordinates and reduces clinical and administrative efforts

▶ Redesigns and shares services among departments and organizations

▶ Strives for internal and external customer satisfaction

▶ Is a core business (functionally and structurally)

Essential Functions of a Integrated Case Management (ICM) System

The general functionality of ICM is that it is a patient-centric, easily accessible, and navigable system. A complete patient profile may be viewed from one location across different diseases and for all care programs and activities. The ability to modify or add disease and condition protocols, care plans, and alerts and reminders is an advantage for care management. ICM facilitates communication and collaboration among the interdisciplinary teams and providers. The point-of-care functions include a patient summary screen that can be customized; a current and complete display of previous care and outcomes; and prebuilt and user-developed documentation tools, templates, and workflows. Decision support is available through access to guidelines and protocols plus the ability to add or change them. Patient self-management captures data about self-care behaviors, and ICM will provide tracking and documentation to the patient. Population management is accomplished using standard formats that can be customized, tracking population and provider panels as well as accommodating different medical conditions. In addition, there are initiatives to track and improve patient health. Finally, the ICM reporting function produces both standard and ad hoc reports at an individual and aggregate level. The reporting function also monitors quality and tracks outcomes.

Potential Risk Factors and Barriers to the Nurse Case Management (NCM) Process

A variety of challenges may occur during the NCM process. These are described as patient, practitioner, and system-level risk factors and barriers. Patient barriers may include:

- Poor attitude
- Memory deficits
- Language
- Literacy
- Cultural beliefs
- Alternative health beliefs
- Poor support
- Pride

- Denial
- Fear or embarrassment
- Side effects
- Religious beliefs
- Inability to "see" results of drug therapy
- Lack of choices
- Cost

How do we address patient risk factors and barriers? Identify strategies and tools to assist in resolution, such as motivational interviewing techniques, utilizing a readiness ruler, a Modified Morisky Scale to educate patients regarding adherence, a My Medication List (National Transitions of Care Coalition, 2009), and the Patient's Bill of Rights during transitions of care.

Provider barriers and risk factors can include the following:

- Practitioners may not know the patient, family, or caregiver.
- Practitioners may not be familiar with patient's, family's, or caregiver's preferences for care.
- Practitioners often are not familiar with the operations of the settings where they transfer patients.
- Sending and receiving practitioners may not communicate critical information.
- Practitioners have no accountability.

What actions are useful to case managers when facing provider risk factors and barriers? Start with a shift from the "discharge concept" to "transfer with continuous management." Many nurse case managers are familiar with the statement "discharge begins at admission"; therefore, transfer planning begins upon or even before admission, during the assessment and planning process. Identify actual or potential barriers early to employ case manager interventions such as community resource referrals. Include the patient's, family's, and caregiver's preferences in the nurse case management plan and alert the provider or practitioner about the support system. Ask the question, "How will you care for yourself when you get home or leave the hospital, rehabilitation facility, or nursing home?" Who is available to assist the patient with activities of daily living and instrumental activities of daily living? There may be a home health aide for personal care with skilled home health visits, but what about shopping, laundry, preparing meals, and transportation? Achieving a safe transition of care is paramount for the nurse case manager. Finally, collaborate with practitioners and providers across settings and levels of care to formulate and execute a common care plan.

System barriers and risk factors are related to healthcare facilities and our healthcare delivery system. Nurse case managers are confronted daily with system barriers as they navigate a fragmented structure to enable patients to transition from one level of care to another. These system barriers include:

► Systems remain in silos

► Communications between practitioners and facilities that are poor or nonexistent

► Care coordinators or points of contact that are not identified

► A lack of accountability on the sending or receiving end of a transition (Coleman, 2003)

How do nurse case managers address these barriers in a fragmented healthcare system? Preferably, healthcare facilities would have interoperable information systems. There are health systems with electronic health records (EHR) and even in this setting, there can be difficulties when the inpatient EHR software is not integrated with the outpatient EHR. Sharing health records is essential for a smooth referral and transition of care. This should be managed via discharge software, encrypted e-mail, a fax with HIPAA statement cover sheet, or even in person, with a hand-off of the health record to the receiving facility. Care plans with common data elements and standardized outcome measures promote understanding of the expected goals and reduce confusion regarding key data, such as demographics and payer information. Administrative buy-in promotes smooth, seamless transfers because the expectations are set by facility management. Informed decision-making allows the patient, family, and caregiver to exercise their autonomy, as opposed to an informed consent process, in which they are instructed in a plan.

Case Simulation: Mr. Garza has heart failure, diabetes, and hypertension. He sees a PCP, cardiologist, and endocrinologist. His prescription list includes more than six medications, plus three over-the-counter medications, prescribed by his various providers. He has Medicare, receives Social Security income, and has a small pension. Mrs. Garza calls the hospital nurse case manager after her husband's most recent cardiology hospitalization, asking if he should continue to take the same medications as before and the new ones. The nurse case manager reviews the discharge instructions and the medication reconciliation document and discovers that two of the medications were rewritten with brand-name labels, but Mrs. Garza asked about them using the generic names. When contacting Mr. and Mrs. Garza, the nurse case manager clarifies the discharge medication list, instructs the patient and his wife which prescriptions to fill, and explains the different labels for the same medications. The Garzas express their appreciation because they budget for their medications and have expressed concern regarding the costs for the brand-name medications. The nurse case manager contacts the outpatient pharmacy that Mr. Garza uses and gives a verbal order for the generic equivalent medication after receiving substitute prescriptions from the discharging provider. Following the conversation with the pharmacy, the nurse case manager contacts the PCP and endocrinology clinics to alert them to Mr. Garza's hospitalization and sends the discharge summary, via fax, to the clinics. Included in the fax is the medication reconciliation document with a reminder to review it at each patient visit. Documentation for this activity includes the patient and family contact, record review, case management interventions, and the patient and family response.

Communicating, collaborating, and facilitating with stakeholders is critical for a successful case manager plan and outcomes; high-quality care; cost-effective outcomes; and patient, family, and caregiver satisfaction. An effective stakeholder team communicates all case management activities in a timely manner and ensures collaboration among team members. The stakeholder team is prepared to continually problem-solve and employs effective conflict resolution techniques, thus enabling them to work productively toward a common goal and in the patient's best interest.

REFERENCES

Advanced Mentoring Healthcare. (2008). Retrieved from www.healthcare.advancedmentoring.com/index.php/FindPage=Difference%20Between%20Precepting%20and%20Mentoring%20and%20ot&LayoutSet=short

Agency for Healthcare Research and Quality. (2011). *AHRQ evidence report.* Retrieved from www.ahrq.gov

Alper, B. S., Hand, J. A., Elliott, S. G., Kinkade, S., Hauan, M. J., Onion, D. K., & Sklar, B. M. (2004). How much effort is needed to keep up with literature relevant for primary care? *Journal of the Medical Library Association, 92*(4), 429–437.

American Nurses Association. (2010). *Nursing scope and standards of practice* (2nd ed.). Silver Spring, MD: Author

Balas, E. A., & Boren, S. A. (2000). *Managing clinical knowledge for healthcare improvement.* Retrieved from www.ihi.org/Knowledge/Pages/Publications/Managing clinicalknowledgefor healthcareimprovement.aspx

Busen, N., & Engebretson, J. (1999). *Mentoring in advanced practice nursing: The use of metaphor in concept exploration.* Retrieved from www.icaap.org

Case Management Society of America. (2006–2007). *Case management adherence guidelines, version 2.* Little Rock, AR: Author.

Case Management Society of America. (2010). *Standards of practice for case management.* Little Rock, AR: Author.

Case Management Society of America. (2012). *Our history.* Retrieved from www.cmsa.org/Home/CMSA/OurHistory/tabid/225/Default.aspx

Cesta, T. G., Tahan, H. A., & Fink, L. A. (2002). *The case manager's survival guide: Winning strategies for clinical practice.* St. Louis, MO: Mosby.

Coleman, E. (2003). *Falling through the cracks: Challenges and opportunities for improving transitional care for persons with continuous complex care needs.* Retrieved from www.caretransitions.org/documents/Falling%20through%20the%20cracks%20-%20JAGS

Covell, D. G., Uman, G. C., & Manning, P. R. (1985). Information needs in office practice: Are they being met? *Annals of Internal Medicine, 103*(4), 596–599.

Edwards, P. (1996). *The specialty practice of rehabilitation nursing: A core curriculum.* Glenview, IL: The Association of Rehabilitation Nurses.

Forcible Figures: J. Bowman. (2008). *Case in practice, leadership supplement.* Retrieved from www.caseinpoint.cmrg.com/cip_200805.pdf

Geissler, E. M. (1994). *Pocket guide to cultural assessment* (2nd ed.). St. Louis, MO: Mosby.

Gilbert, R., Salanti, G., Harden, M., & See, S. (2005). Infant sleeping position and the sudden infant death syndrome: Systematic review of observational studies and historical review of recommendations from 1940 to 2002. *International Journal of Epidemiology, 34*(4), 874–887.

Henry J. Kaiser Family Foundation, The. (2012). *Trends in health care costs and spending.* Retrieved from http://www.kff.org/insurance/upload/7692.pdf

Hicks, T. (2007). *Seven steps for effective problem solving in the workplace.* Retrieved from http://www.mediate.com/articles/thicks.cfm

Howe, R. (2005). *The disease manager's handbook.* Sudbury, MA: Jones & Bartlett.

Insignia Health. (2012). *Patient activation measure*. Retrieved from www.insigniahealth.com/solutions/patient-activation-measure

Karthol, R. G., Perez, R., & Cohen, C. (2010). *The integrated case management manual*. New York. Springer Publishing.

Klainberg, M., Holzemer, S., Leonard, M., & Arnold, J. (1998). *Community health nursing: An alliance for health*. New York: McGraw-Hill.

Llewellyn, A., & Leonard, M. (2009). *Nursing case management review and resource manual* (3rd ed.). Silver Spring, MD: American Nurses Credentialing Center.

McDonough, M. (2011). *Explaining Pareto's 80/20 rule*. Retrieved from www.brighthub.com/office//project-management/articles/65152.aspx

Medscape. (2011). *State CE requirements for nurses*. Retrieved from www.medscape.org/public/nursecestaterequirements

Moriskey, D. E., Green, L. W., & Seeds, S. G. (1986). Concurrent and predictive validity of a self-reported measure of medication adherence. *Medical Care, 24*, 67–74.

National Center for Chronic Disease Prevention and Health Promotion. (2008). *About chronic disease*. Retrieved from www.cdc.gov/nccdphp/about.htm

National Institutes of Health. (1996). *Coping with chronic illness* (Patient information publication). Bethesda, MD: Warren Grant Magnuson Clinical Center.

National Transitions of Care Coalition. (2009). *Improving transitions of care: Hospital to home*. Retrieved from www.ntocc.org/Portals/0/PDF/Resources/ImplementationPlans_Hospital to Home.pdf

Peplau, H. (1974). Is healthcare a right? *Image: Journal of Nursing Scholarship, 7*(1), 4–10.

Prochaska, J. O., & Prochaska, J. M. (1999). Helping cure health care systems: Changing minds and behaviour. *Disease Management & Health Outcomes, 6*(6), 335–341.

QualityMetric. (2012). *SF-36 and SF-12*. Retrieved from www.sf-36.org/tools

Ringel, M. (1998). Implementing health status measurements. *Medical Management Newsletter, 6*(1), 1–4.

Sabate, E. (Ed.) (2003). *Adherence to long-term therapies: Evidence for action*. Geneva, Switzerland: World Health Organization.

Schmidt, N., & Brown, J. (2008). *Evidence-based practice for nurses: Appraisal and application of research*. Sudbury, MA: Jones & Bartlett Learning.

United States Preventive Task Force (USPSTF). (2011). *Pocket guide to clinical preventative services, 2010-2011*. Retrieved from www.uspreventiveservicetaskforce.org/index

Zenger, J. H., & Folkman, J. (2002). *The extraordinary leader: Turning good managers into great leaders*. Columbus, OH: McGraw-Hill Professional.

CHAPTER 3

RESOURCE MANAGEMENT

> **"**Can anyone remember when times were not difficult and money was not *scarce.***"**
> —*Ralph Waldo Emerson*

In today's world, there are two major areas of concern: one is the economy and the other is health care. It is important for case managers to be aware of their patients' economic status, including whether or not they are insured, and if they are insured, what is covered in their insurance benefit package. Case managers should also be familiar with the new Patient Protection and Affordable Care Act (PPACA). On March 23, 2010, the president signed a comprehensive health reform bill, PPACA, into law. This legislation focuses on provisions to expand coverage, control healthcare costs, and improve the healthcare delivery system. It contains many provisions that the case manager should be aware of that are discussed in detail in Chapter 5.

One of the key functions case managers strive to achieve is ensuring that patients and their families have the tools and resources they need to manage their conditions. Doing so allows them to gain confidence, regain control of their lives, and move toward self-management, which is one of the ultimate goals of the process of case management.

As we learned in Chapter 2, identification of patients at risk is the first step in the case management process. Once the patients are identified, the case manager begins her or his assessment of the patient, working within an integrated model of care framework. This assessment allows the case manager to assess the patient's behavior and learn about barriers and unmet needs that may be causing problems in his or her life.

To understand human behavior and needs, we can look to the noted theorist, Abraham Maslow, whose work found that until people satisfy their lower needs, starting with survival, they cannot move forward through the other needs required to attain their full potential. Maslow presents a hierarchy of needs pyramid, which can be divided into basic (or deficiency) needs (e.g., physiological, safety, love, esteem) and growth needs (cognitive, aesthetics, self-actualization). One must satisfy lower-level basic needs before progressing to meet higher-level growth needs. Once these needs have been reasonably satisfied, one may be able to reach the highest level, called "self-actualization" (Mcleod, 2007).

Resource Management

Taking the time to understand where a patient is in his or her life and ensuring that his or her basic needs are met is the basis of resource management. *Resource management* is defined as the process of identifying, confirming, coordinating, and negotiating resources to meet the individual needs of a person (Bower & Falk, 1996). It is a goal-oriented approach that requires extensive coordination and is an integral part of each step in the case management process.

As part of the assessment process, the case manager uses all of his or her senses to understand barriers to wellness and the needs of the patient. Depending on these findings, securing appropriate resources can range from a simple phone call to an ongoing research project. Services can include connecting a patient to a primary care medical home; referring a patient with a fractured ankle to an orthopedic surgeon because he or she has recently relocated and has not yet established a relationship with a primary care provider; assisting a patient with diabetes who has lost healthcare coverage to secure funding for insulin, syringes, and other diabetic supplies; securing emergency housing for a family that is homeless; or calling protective services for a woman who has been abused, among other activities. As is evident, resource management encompasses a wide range of activities, and can be both stressful and time-consuming. Learning to balance time spent on resource management with other components of the case management process is important. Having a reliable list of resources and current community services can reduce stress and maximize efficiency. Networking with fellow case managers and other members of the healthcare team adds to options case managers can tap into when working with complicated patients. As case managers mature in their roles, they become savvier in navigating the system and more creative in their abilities to effectively and efficiently meet the needs of their patient.

REVIEW CRITERIA

Although case managers have spent years distinguishing themselves from utilization review nurses, utilization management remains an important part of the case management process. The documented scarcity of healthcare resources in the United States has created a great demand for resource management skills. This scarcity and advances in medical technology and an aging population are creating new challenges for healthcare organizations as they struggle to improve quality and become more efficient. These challenges call for managing care in a way that fosters evidence-based practice and ensures patient safety while controlling costs.

The nurse case manager cannot rely on yesterday's theories and clinical expectations. Therefore, he or she must look to care coordination tools that have evolving abilities to meet clinical challenges, apply clinical research, and use technologies to enhance health and humanity. The following are two decision support tools that are used extensively in the field to assist nurse case managers in their roles: Milliman Care Guidelines and InterQual. Naturally, these tools do not replace appropriate training for nurse case managers nor their sound clinical judgment, but stand as evidence-based guidelines on which case managers can base their care coordination decisions.

Milliman Care Guidelines

This series of evidence-based guidelines serves as a tool that describes best practices for treating common conditions and delivering chronic care and behavioral health services in a variety of settings—inpatient, ambulatory care, patient's home, doctor's office, and so forth. These clinical tools, which are designed to be concise, actionable, and measurable, assist case managers in providing high-quality care by reducing inappropriate care—either underuse or overuse—and the misuse of healthcare resources.

The Milliman Care Guidelines are just that, guidelines that are clear and direct. They are not a prescription, a decision tree, or a set of rules for the practice of medicine. They are a snapshot of what is possible and what is actually being done. They incorporate nationally recognized quality measures and patient education tools. They are planning tools designed to assist the case manager when coordinating patient care and anticipating the patient's needs (Milliman, 2012).

InterQual™

InterQual products are clinical decision support tools used in determining when and how a patient progresses through the continuum of care. They help healthcare organizations facilitate quality of care and clinical resource utilization by providing objective criteria based on well-researched scientific knowledge and real-world clinical experience to assess the appropriate care for individual patients.

This tool can help the nurse case manager apply evidence-based information consistently, promote appropriate care, improve care coordination and provider collaboration, manage administration of biotech drugs, and address fraud and abuse.

These tools also help case managers to

► Explore the relationships among utilization, case, and disease management;

► Integrate care management processes and understand the relevance of corresponding outcomes;

► Meet regulatory and accreditation guidelines and goals;

► Understand legal liability and ethical considerations, as well as the impact of legislation, and

► Identify financial risk to meet the current demand for balanced cost and quality (McKesson, 2012).

Every case manager struggles with the challenge of how to best leverage limited dollars to have the greatest impact on health and costs. Therefore, tools that help case managers integrate utilization, case, and disease management efforts, as well as good communication among all the stakeholders, serve them well.

Case Simulation: A nurse case manager working for a managed care organization identifies a member as a candidate for case management services through the health plan's daily inpatient census. The patient living with diabetes had fallen at home and broken her hip. The plan case manager has been communicating with the hospital case manager, and together they coordinated the patient's care as she made the transition from the hospital to an acute rehabilitation facility and then to outpatient physical therapy in her home. The plan case manager also monitored and gave approval for all of the patient's services, durable medical equipment, medications, and so on.

An important part of the case management process is the coordination and reconciliation of the patient's medications. The patient switched from one blood pressure medication to another and her cholesterol-lowering medication dosage also changed while she was in the hospital. The provider felt the patient did very well on these new medications and her tolerance was good. Therefore, he wrote prescriptions for these new medications and gave them to the discharge nurse to give to the patient upon hospital discharge.

The plan case manager approved the in-home physical therapy three times a week for 8 weeks. She approved an evaluation by a home care nurse, who would also conduct a medication reconciliation and ensure that the patient understood her new medication regimen and filled her new prescriptions. The visiting nurse reported back to the plan case manager that the patient was doing well and was safe in her home, but that she needed one more visit from the nurse to ensure medication compliance. The plan case manager approved the extra nursing visit.

After a period of a few weeks, the plan case manager noticed that progress notes from the physical therapist had not been received as requested. She called the therapist; he was happy to give the case manager an update and promised to send the notes. The following week the therapist asked for approval of 12 more visits—4 additional weeks of therapy. When the plan case manager read the progress notes, she realized that the notes did not reflect the conversation she had had with the therapist. In fact, the notes read as though there was no progress being made by the patient in the last 2 weeks, or 6 visits. The plan case manager referred to the Milliman Care Guidelines and saw that continued services are not warranted when there has been no documentation of continuous improvement. She called the therapist to explain the criteria and asked that he make alternative plans for an in-home self-directed exercise program. She also arranged for the patient to follow up with her primary care provider in 2 weeks. So that the therapist could accomplish these interventions, the case manager approved four more physical therapy sessions—two visits a week for 2 weeks. The case manager is confident in her decision because it was based on these nationally accepted evidence-based clinical guidelines.

The therapist instructed the patient and was confident that the patient understood the plan of care. The therapist developed a self-administered exercise program for the patient to follow and asked the patient to do a return demonstration of the exercises. The patient was also able to list signs and symptoms of something gone awry. The therapist told the patient he would follow up with her in a week to see how she was doing and confirm that the patient had made a follow-up appointment with the doctor.

In this scenario, the patient is receiving the appropriate care in the appropriate setting at the appropriate cost. Everyone, including the healthcare system, wins.

UTILIZATION MANAGEMENT

Utilization management (UM) is the evaluation of the appropriateness of the medical treatment and of the efficiency of healthcare services, procedures, and resources. The evaluation is based on established clinical criteria or guidelines under the requirements of the patient's individual benefit plan. Utilization management differs from utilization review (UR) in that it is a forward-looking process intended to manage healthcare resources efficiently and cost-effectively. Utilization review, on the other hand, is performed to ensure that the patient's "five rights" are observed: the patient receives the *right* services at the *right* time delivered by the *right* provider in the *right* setting for the *right* cost. There are three components of utilization review—preauthorization, concurrent, and retrospective.

Today, the healthcare industry realizes that focusing solely on the cost of care is not the most efficient way to manage resources or ensure quality and continuity of care. Thus, the focus of UR has broadened to focus more attention on utilization management of resources, which includes looking at the type of care being provided and ensuring that evidence-based criteria to support decisions, policies for appropriate resource allocation, and quality measure mechanisms are all in place.

In many organizations, utilization management is considered a "trigger" into case management. Through the use of integrated IT tools, patients who have repeat admissions, major setbacks to their care, or social problems that impede adherence or compliance can be triaged by the UM nurse specialist into case management services. Once a patient is identified, the case manager performs an assessment to understand the patient's needs and develops an individualized care plan that holistically addresses barriers to care. The ability to ensure this collaboration has evolved further with the development of predictive modeling programs (discussed in Chapter 4) and risk stratification tools. The result is earlier identification of those at risk and implementation of interventions to allow for early and effective management.

As the population ages, thanks to scientific advances that allow people to live longer, preventing and managing chronic illnesses and complications inherent in older populations becomes more critical. The emergence of disease management programs has enabled medical professionals to better understand and effectively control aspects of care through more specific interventions for these disease processes. Blending the principles of disease management, utilization management, and case management provides payers and providers with a three-pronged approach to patient care management across the continuum of life (Carneal, 2000). This blending continues to evolve over time. In order to keep pace, case managers and other healthcare professionals are challenged to maintain and enhance clinical competencies, as well as to develop new patient education strategies regarding the importance of behavior modification and taking more active roles in healthcare decisions.

Authorization and Certification

Preauthorization Review

Preauthorization or preadmission review is performed before a service is started or a product is purchased. It is used to determine the actual need for a patient's admission or treatment as outlined by a specific provider.

Case Simulations: A 55-year-old female with chronic pain is told she needs a hip replacement because of osteoarthritis. The managed care organization's guidelines state that a second opinion for all patients under the age of 65 receiving hip replacements is required. The rationale for this is that, because of the cost of hip replacements, the managed care organization wants to ensure that all conservative measures have been exhausted prior to authorizing a hip replacement.

Once the denial is rendered, the patient and provider are notified by the UM department's preadmission nurse of the decision made by the medical director who reviewed the claim. They are given the recommendation of either seeking a second opinion by an orthopedic surgeon elsewhere in the network, or consulting with her provider for alternative treatment. The patient decides to get a second opinion.

When a denial is made, it is required that the provider and patient be notified and given the clinical rationale for the denial, as well as their rights to appeal the decision. Many times, the denial is made because of lack of information. Providing additional information allows the managed care team to review the claim again to see if the information submitted meets the clinical criteria. However, if the provider and patient feel that the information sufficiently met the clinical criteria, they have the right to appeal the decision.

Concurrent Review

Concurrent review is a process used to document the continuation of a service and level of care a patient may be receiving, such as a continued hospital stay or continuation of rehabilitation. Concurrent reviews occur while services are ongoing to ensure that the setting and care still meet the clinical criteria for the patient's condition.

Concurrent reviews are done according to specific time frames on the basis of the patient's condition. The UM nurse, as part of the authorization process, provides the length of time or the number of services that payment is approved for and when the next review is scheduled. On the basis of this, the provider prepares the report necessary to justify the claim or move, or discharge the patient to a lower level of care. The provider is challenged to support the level of care requested with adequate documentation that complies with the clinical criteria. If a denial is made, the managed care organization must supply both provider and patient with the clinical review criteria so that they understand how the decision was made and provide clinical rationale to support the decision.

Case Simulation: A patient in a rehabilitation facility for therapy related to a head injury is initially approved for a 2-week period. The rehabilitation case manager responsible for providing an update to the managed care organization's UM department must show the progress or lack of progress the patient has made from one review cycle to the next, and explain the goals the team feels the patient can achieve with continued therapy. Depending on the outcome of the case manager's report, the team will be informed and the plan of care will be continued, or an alternative plan may need to be developed. If the continued stay is denied, the managed care organization will give the rationale for the denial and what criteria were used to make the decision. Many times, the team agrees with the decision and will discharge the patient or move the patient to a lower level of care. If the team feels strongly that the patient should remain at the current level of care, however, an appeal is made and additional clinical data to support the request are provided to the managed care organization according to the appeal process. Detailed documentation regarding all discussions is incorporated into the patient's chart.

Two examples of well-known clinical criteria that managed care organizations, as well as providers, use include InterQual and Milliman Care Guidelines. These criteria are described earlier in this chapter. Many organizations develop their own clinical guidelines with the input from their medical teams and specialists within their networks. Because clinical criteria change as a result of advances in science and technology, it is recommended that clinical guidelines be reviewed on an annual basis to ensure they are up to date with the latest evidence.

Retrospective Review

A retrospective review is performed after care or service is provided. Retrospective reviews can be viewed as part of the continuous quality improvement process that both the provider and the payer use to improve services.

Many managed care organizations have reduced or eliminated the precertification process but look retrospectively to see how providers have managed patient care over time. If a provider is seen as an outlier (one who either under- or overutilizes services) when measured against peers, the managed care organization can use its national retrospective claims data to demonstrate how the provider compares with his or her peers who have similar patients. This process has led to improvement in practice and has also given validation to the use of evidence-based medicine to guide practice. Organizations that use these tools as comparison markers or benchmarks in retrospective review must remember that they are meant to be guides, not clinical decision-makers. Outlier decisions made by clinicians during a patient's course of care may have valid reasoning based upon a difficult case or unusual circumstances. Retrospective review paints a picture of what occurred, and allows both payers and providers to determine potential changes that can be made to promote continuous quality improvement.

Benefits of Coverage

Healthcare reimbursement systems vary greatly in benefit design and coverage. These specifics are included in member handbooks when coverage begins. Utilization managers, case managers, and providers alike can no longer claim ignorance regarding the covered benefits of a specific payer; all they need do is look to these handbooks or go online to familiarize themselves with their patients' benefit plans, rules, and limitations. If a request for benefit information is made, the payer is obligated to provide that information in a timely manner; otherwise, a grievance can be filed.

As discussed in the previous section, the goal of utilization management is to meet an individual's healthcare needs via appropriate use of resources. Assuming that a patient has health insurance, it is important for the utilization manager, case manager, or both to determine the patient's benefits in order to verify if the payer covers the plan of care. The type of benefit plan the patient has determines the scope of services and benefit coverage that apply. Many times, authorization is needed before ordering services or products.

Because of rising healthcare premiums, many employers switch plans frequently to save dollars. Keeping up with various benefit packages is challenging for even the savviest person. Today, many plans have restrictions on products, services, and formularies, so understanding the benefit plan is important when developing and implementing the plan of care.

Case Simulation: *A provider sends a patient for lab tests to a noncontracted laboratory. The patient goes to the diagnostic lab and has the lab work performed. Subsequently, the patient receives a bill from the lab stating that the managed care plan has denied payment for the cost of the lab services performed because the laboratory was not a contracted network provider for the plan. The patient calls the laboratory billing department thinking a mistake has occurred. The billing department advises the patient to call the managed care plan to discuss billing questions. The customer service representative at the managed care organization checks the list of network providers and informs the patient that he went to a lab that was out of network. The patient argues that he went to the lab that his provider's nurse instructed him to go to. The managed care plan's customer service representative informs the patient that he—not the referring provider—is ultimately responsible for knowing his benefit plan and which providers are in the network. This exchange immediately sets up an adversarial situation among the patient, the payer, and the provider. The outcome is that the patient is responsible for the total bill.*

Many times, patients do not realize that it is necessary to use a network provider for diagnostic tests, when seeing a physician, or if undergoing therapy. Because many providers participate in multiple plans and use various diagnostic labs within those networks, referring a patient to the wrong lab can easily occur. Utilization managers, case managers, and healthcare providers have a responsibility to verify benefits for all procedures and services as part of the utilization process. Proactively educating the patient and the family to become familiar with the guidelines of their insurance policy is important because the patient can be held financially responsible for charges. It should be noted that most states do not allow balance billing for Medicaid beneficiaries.

Contract Interpretation and Negotiations

Insurance policies are legal contracts that detail the scope of services and benefits provided within a policy. Managed care organizations have a responsibility to inform enrollees what their policies include and any exclusions to the benefits package. When a patient requires a procedure or a service that is not covered as part of his or her benefit plan, the case manager can try to negotiate with the carrier by providing information that clearly shows why an uncovered service should be allowed as an exception to the plan. An important piece of information to go with this documentation is a cost–benefit analysis that shows what the cost would be if the service were covered and what the expected outcome would be as a result of the exception versus what the current situation is. This information allows managed care plans to make informed decisions. If an exception to the policy is granted, the case manager should document the exception and keep the insurer updated on the patient's progress.

On the other hand, if an exception is not granted, but the provider feels that the service is needed, then he or she has the responsibility to provide the service. It is important to remember that the denial the payer is rendering is for payment of the service, not for the service itself.

It is always better to err on the side of the patient and have a good outcome than to not provide a needed service on the basis of a payment decision. Otherwise, serious problems could result. Case managers and providers must not rely solely on the benefit plan to meet the needs of the patient, but on the patient's current status to ensure that progress is being made. Also, as reviewed earlier in this chapter, community resources might be available to meet the individual needs of the patient, when there are no benefits to cover necessary services.

Transitions of Care

Transitions of care refers to the movement of the patient from one setting or level of care to another or the movement of the patient between providers. Case managers should realize that the last thing most people want to concern themselves with when they or their loved ones are dealing with a health issue is ensuring effective communication among their healthcare team—doctors, nurses, social workers, and other healthcare providers. However, it is poor communication between well-intentioned professionals and an expectation that patients themselves will remember and relate critical information that can lead to dangerous and even life-threatening situations (National Transitions of Care Coalition, 2011).

Case managers believe patients are at the center of care and can and should play an active role in their care. By being a partner in their own health care, patients can make a difference. However, case managers also realize that when patients and their family or caregivers are in the midst of a health situation, they may become anxious and unable to retain important information given to them or be nervous about asking their provider questions they may have. This is where case managers can help. One can say that transitions of care offer the case manager opportunities to educate patients and the family or caregiver and introduce them to tools that will assist them with safe transitions of care. A great resource for the case manager is the The National Transitions of Care Coalition. This coalition has developed may tools to assist patients, family, caregivers, providers, and case managers with safe transitions. These tools are free and available on their Web site: www.NTOCC.org.

Discharge Planning

Discharge planning is the process of assessing the care needs of a patient to ensure that the transition to the next level of care is appropriate and safe, with the necessary services in place to meet the needs of the patient. The most important element of successful discharge planning is ensuring a safe discharge. Another aspect of discharge planning is the education of the patient and the family to ensure they understand discharge instructions, the medication regimen, and the importance of doing a medication reconciliation when they return home in order to have a handle on the steps they need to take once they leave the facility, and to feel comfortable with equipment they may be required to use once discharged. Case managers involved in discharge planning should make a follow-up call to ensure that all required aspects of the plan of care are in place and that the patient and family are coping well. If the patient is discharged home, it is important to have a scheduled follow-up visit with his or her primary care provider. This small detail helps identify and address problems early on and allows the case manager to ensure his or her role throughout the transition of care is complete. Lastly, documentation of all steps of the discharge plan is essential.

Denials and Appeals Process

Although managed care has been difficult for many providers and consumers to understand and adapt to over the years, the managed care climate has definitely improved. Difficulties in the past were largely attributed to the rules and regulations implemented by managed care organizations, which were viewed as roadblocks to prevent access to needed medical care. The philosophy of managed care is to provide members access to care in a timely and cost-effective manner. To comply with this philosophy, managed care organizations approve services that meet evidence-based criteria.

Providers need to understand this and provide documentation to demonstrate how the recommended services are supported by evidence. If the UM department of a managed care organization denies an admission, a treatment, or a procedure, the provider and the patient have a right to "due process" and can appeal that decision. Most states, as well as the accreditation bodies that accredit managed care organizations, require managed care organizations to have formal processes and timelines in place to inform patients and providers about their rights concerning the denials and the appeals process.

Once a denial is rendered, the provider has the right to appeal the decision and provide additional documentation to show why payment should be reconsidered. It is important to know that only physicians can deny services. Utilization management nurses do not have the authority to deny claims. Their role is to collect the data, verify that the request meets clinical criteria, and ensure that the patient has a benefit to cover the request. If there are questions regarding benefits or if the claim does not meet medical criteria used, the claim is turned over to the medical director, who makes the final decision.

Each managed care organization has a department dedicated to handling appeals and grievances, as well as policy and procedures to guide the process. Understanding the language regarding appeals and grievances is important to the patient and the family or caregiver. An appeal is a formal method of lodging a disagreement over a claim payment or benefit denial. Once an appeal is filed, the managed care organization is obligated to answer the appeal within a certain period of time. If the request is denied, but a provider feels there is an urgent need for treatment, the provider can make the appeal an urgent request so that the process can be expedited. This is called an *expedited appeal*.

When appealing a claim, all benefit information and medical documentation supporting the medical necessity for the service or procedure must be provided. Many times, the medical director will consult with the provider to understand the need for the claim. As a result of these peer-to-peer discussions, the denial may be overturned because the medical director has a better understanding of the treating provider's rationale. All efforts, specific timelines, and conversations must be documented by both the provider case manager and the managed care utilization nurse. After all information is reviewed and if the denial is upheld, the patient and the provider are notified in writing that the denial has been made, what the clinical criteria used to make the decision were, and the right to appeal the decision.

Once an appeal is made, the managed care organization must have the claim reviewed by a physician who is of the same specialty as the requested service and not the person who made the original decision. To meet this requirement, many managed care organizations retain independent review organizations. The independent review physician receives all of the documentation available on the claim, performs a review of the material against the current clinical evidence, and renders a decision. The specialist also takes the opportunity to speak with the treating physician to clarify any questions and shape his or her viewpoint. Once a decision is made, the provider and the patient are notified in writing. If the decision is in favor of the claim, the payer must cover the claim. If the specialist upholds the denial decision, then the payer does not need to pay the claim, and the provider will develop an alternative plan. In some states, the provider and the patient may ask for a *fair hearing*.

In addition to the appeals process, managed care organizations are required to set up a process in which providers and patients are able to voice complaints or grievances. A *grievance* is a formal method of lodging a complaint with the managed care organization. A grievance can be filed by the managed care organization itself against a network provider; by the network provider against the managed care organization; or by a patient regarding the managed care organization, the network provider, or both. Grievances are filed by the managed care member or provider when there is a delay in care or another care-related issue. Filing a written grievance gives the managed care organization a formal opportunity to address the problem and rectify the situation. If a provider or a member takes the time to file a grievance, the managed care organization will follow all prescribed policies and procedures regarding processes and timelines for handling the grievance.

External Review

If a patient receives an adverse benefit determination, he or she also has the right to request an external review of the claim. In most states, this request is handled by the department of insurance and is handled outside of the insurance company that issued the denial. In cases where time is of the essence, a case many be referred to the state for an expedited review.

A claimant may make a written or oral request for an expedited external review with the examiner when the claimant receives:

> An adverse benefit determination if the adverse benefit determination involves a medical condition of the claimant for which the time frame for completion of an expedited internal appeal under the interim final regulations would seriously jeopardize the life or health of the claimant or would jeopardize the claimant's ability to regain maximum function and the claimant has filed a request for an expedited internal appeal, or an adverse benefit determination if the adverse benefit determination concerns an admission, availability of care, continued stay, or health care item or service for which the claimant received services, but has not been discharged from a facility, and the claimant has filed a request for an expedited internal appeal; or

> A final internal adverse benefit determination, if the claimant has a medical condition where the time frame for completion of a standard external review would seriously jeopardize the life or health of the claimant or would jeopardize the claimant's ability to regain maximum function, or if the final internal adverse benefit determination concerns an admission, availability of care, continued stay, or health care item or service for which the claimant received services, but has not been discharged from a facility. (U.S. Department of Health and Human Services, 2010)

LEVEL OF CARE OPTIONS

Following is an overview of the various levels of care settings that exist in the current healthcare system and a description of the functions performed by the case managers who work in these settings. To help guide decision-making regarding level of care, case managers should remember the essence of case management: *It is the role of the case manager to ensure patients receive safe, high-quality, evidence-based care in the least restrictive setting, and at the most appropriate time for the most cost-effective price.* Keeping this saying in mind will help case managers guide practice, ensure appropriate resources, and contain escalating healthcare costs.

Acute Care

Acute care hospitals in the United States represent the largest segment of healthcare settings. Hospitals and related physician expenditures traditionally account for the majority of healthcare spending. In 2010, $814.0 billion spent on health care was attributed to hospital spending (U.S. Department of Health & Human Services, 2012). Because of the rising costs of healthcare spending, a radical redesign has been imposed on all aspects of the healthcare system, with the acute care setting being hardest hit. The government, payers, and accrediting organizations have imposed many rules and regulations that focus on improving efficiency and appropriateness of services. Funding to hospitals has been decreased, which has caused hospital administrators and chief financial officers to struggle for ways to comply yet remain profitable. Today, it is not easy to get admitted to a hospital. For a patient to be admitted, the treating provider must provide documentation based on clinical criteria that the patient meets the requirements for admission and the level of care requested.

The purpose of the acute care setting is to diagnose and treat those who are too sick to have procedures and treatments performed in the outpatient setting. Clear documentation that includes medical necessity for testing and procedures is needed from the healthcare team. This information is submitted to payers to evaluate whether the procedures and care requested meet the required criteria. The case manager who works in the acute care setting is responsible for obtaining this information from the treating physicians and, once approved, ensuring that procedures are performed in a timely manner and that results are obtained and interpreted promptly so the healthcare team can determine the next step in the plan of care.

The duties that case managers perform differ from setting to setting, according to the size and philosophy of the healthcare institution. Many acute care settings have sophisticated case management programs that address all aspects of the delivery of care, while other settings are less complex and may focus only on specific functions, such as discharge planning or utilization review. Regardless of the role, the case manager is charged with making sure that the necessary information is obtained so that decisions can be made in an efficient manner. The emphasis on appropriate utilization of services and cost containment continues as a high priority in all acute care hospitals. Many payer organizations send external case managers into the acute care setting to work collaboratively with the acute care team and assist with appropriate resource management.

Acute care case managers are charged with proactively identifying patients who do not meet specific criteria or who have social or financial problems that cause them to have extended or frequent stays. Once obstacles are identified, the case manager can begin to address the needs of the patient, the family, or both by implementing an individualized plan of care. Professionals who practice as acute care case managers usually are nurses and social workers. Many organizations use the combined skills of both professions to effectively meet the needs of the population served through an integrated model of care.

Once a patient is stabilized, arrangements are made for the patient to move to a lesser level of care. For most patients, this could be a move to an acute rehabilitation facility, a subacute facility, or home. It is the responsibility of the discharging facility to document the rationale when a patient is moved from one setting to another. If the patient is going to another facility, the case manager or discharge planner is responsible for ensuring that the transfer is performed in a safe and efficient manner and that the patient is medically stable and agrees to the plan of care. A physician must be willing to accept the patient at the receiving facility and follow the patient in the new setting. To make this transition of care as safe and effective as possible, a report is given to the receiving facility concerning the current status and the ongoing needs of the patient. Once this information is obtained and appropriate papers are signed, a copy of the entire medical record is sent with the patient so that the receiving facility has all the information on what occurred in the acute care setting to provide ongoing care. The case manager or the discharge nurse should be available for any questions that arise as a result of the transfer.

Case Simulation: A 56-year-old man with renal failure, diabetes, chronic obstructive pulmonary disease, and hypertension has been hospitalized on a medical ICU. He has needed continued ventilation via trach and ongoing dialysis. His funding is Medicare and a Medigap plan with a commercial product. The critical care team believes he will be weaned and be able to return home after continued medical care and physical rehabilitation. Long-term acute care (LTAC) appears to be the appropriate level of care, with the medically complex needs plus therapies. Physical therapy, speech–language pathology, and occupational therapy evaluations are ordered. The case manager meets with the patient and family to discuss LTAC options; they choose a facility near the hospital and plan to tour the LTAC later that day. A referral packet is prepared for the LTAC liaison nurse, who will evaluate the patient within 2 hours. The case manager notifies the multidisciplinary team of the LTAC plan and evaluation so that their recommendations are documented for the LTAC evaluation. The case manager meets with the patient, the family, and the LTAC liaison to perform introductions, answer any questions, and offer the referral packet. After an hour, the LTAC nurse liaison informs the case manager that she is contacting the LTAC admissions staff for approval and appropriate bed availability. The patient is approved, and a transfer plan is agreed upon for the next day. A discharge summary is requested from the provider by the case manager, as well as an updated nursing assessment, flowsheet, medication list, and dialysis needs. The respiratory therapist provides current vent settings. Ambulance transport, with vent and ACLS crew, is secured for transport at 10 a.m. the next day. The family returns from their LTAC tour and reports that they are pleased with the facility and services. The patient and family sign the consent for transfer; the family will meet the patient at the LTAC the next day. The case manager completes the transfer documentation, communicates with the LTAC nurse liaison for the transport time, and delivers the completed transfer packet to the transfer center. The following day, the case manager confirms the transport, notifies the nursing staff to call report, and ensures the completed discharge summary is faxed to the LTAC. Once the ambulance arrives, the case manager contacts the LTAC case manager to offer information on family members and availability to discuss the patient once LTAC case management assessment is completed.

Rehabilitation

The rehabilitation setting is the venue where many patients receive care after an injury or an illness that affects their ability to care for themselves, including complications or deficits that affect activities of daily living. Patients who suffer from a cerebral vascular accident, spinal cord injury, traumatic brain injury, amputation, or other illnesses or injuries can benefit from a stay in a rehabilitation setting. Rehabilitation facilities have specialized staff who address the physical, functional, and psychological areas affected by a catastrophic injury or illness. Many rehabilitation facilities elect to meet strict criteria set by the Commission on Accreditation of Rehabilitation Facilities (CARF), which ensures that the facility meets specific standards for safe and effective services.

Rehabilitation can be performed in an inpatient setting, a transitional care setting, an outpatient setting, or at home. Each setting has specific criteria, and the rehabilitation team, led by physiatrists, sets goals, designs the treatment plan, assigns the level of care where treatment is performed, sets time frames for the rehabilitation program, tracks the patient's progress, and makes recommendations regarding the discharge plan. The case manager working in the rehabilitation setting is traditionally a specialist in rehabilitation.

Case Simulation: A 72-year-old widow fell at home and sustained a fractured pelvis. The patient was seen in the emergency department and admitted to the hospital for stabilization. After 4 days, the orthopedic physician recommended discharge to an acute rehabilitation hospital to reteach the patient how to walk. Arrangements were made with the physiatrist at a local rehabilitation center that accepted the patient. Once a bed was available for the patient, she was informed of the move and agreed. The acute care case manager began the process of preparing for the move. She requested a copy of the medical record; set up transportation; and communicated with the patient, the patient's family, and the receiving facility. The patient was transferred to the facility, where she received physical therapy to regain strength, learn how to transfer her weight, and then eventually walk. She began to regain her self-confidence, which was lost following the fall. After 3 weeks, the patient was able to ambulate using a walker and was ready for discharge to home.

Home Care

Patients are now being sent home with complicated medical problems and expected to manage independently for the most part under the direction of their families and caregivers. Case managers and discharge planners must be cautious when discharging a patient to home, and ensure that the family is prepared to safely handle the needs of the patient. To assist with this challenge, many payers contract with home care agencies in their networks to evaluate patients and families so that when the discharge date arrives, the patient and family are ready. The desired outcome is that the patient is able to receive the necessary care at home in a safe and cost-effective manner. The needs of the patient determine the level of care required.

Case Simulation: A case manager coordinating the discharge plan for a ventilator-dependent patient to go home works with an experienced high-tech home care agency to facilitate care for the patient and education and support for the family. This specialized home care agency has professionals with expertise and appropriate credentials to provide both the high-tech nursing and the high-tech respiratory care to meet the patient's needs.

The key to understanding the needs of individual patients as they make the transition from the inpatient setting to the home setting, and of their families or caregivers, is to ensure that a comprehensive assessment is completed using an interdisciplinary team approach. Another key component to a successful transition is education. It helps prepare patients and family members for the return home.

In long-term cases, it is particularly important that attention be paid to the caregiver because this role is difficult and often overlooked. The home care case manager must advocate with the payer and, many times, with members of the patient's family, to ensure that respite care is incorporated into the treatment plan to prevent burnout of the family or caregiver.

Hospice

Hospice care is considered when a chronic condition or an injury is likely to result in death in the "near" future, and the patient does not want aggressive treatment that will prolong life.

Today, it is required that every patient who enters a healthcare setting be asked about advance directives. Advance directives give people a way to communicate how they want to be treated when end of life is approaching. Advance directives must be recognized and respected by the healthcare team. Education of consumers as to how advance directives are used is also important if unnecessary and unwanted procedures are to be prevented per the patient's wishes. Patients should be encouraged to bring a copy of their advance directives with them each time they are admitted to a facility. They should also supply a copy of their advance directives to their primary care providers. Advance directives are covered in more depth in Chapter 5.

Consulting with hospice care professionals is one way the case manager can help the patient and family or caregiver prepare for end-of-life care. The current focus of hospice has shifted from looking at the patient whose death is imminent to working earlier with patients who have progressive chronic illness, such as chronic obstructive pulmonary disease or cancer, to address end-of-life care. Hospice can assist both patients and family or caregivers in preparing for death with dignity and respect. Hospice can be provided in an inpatient setting or in the home, depending on the needs of the patient.

Private-Duty Nursing

Private-duty nursing is implemented in situations when the patient requires one-on-one care. Today, because of the nursing shortage, many families and caregivers are using private-duty nurses to help care for family members while in the hospital. In this scenario, insurance companies do not typically compensate them for the cost of private-duty nursing because it is the family's choice. Another area of focus for private-duty nursing is in the home when a child or an adult who is impaired by a catastrophic event or chronic illness requires extensive nursing care.

Case Simulation: A child who survived a near-drowning is left in a persistent vegetative state and requires 24-hour care to feed, suction, bathe, and provide all the needed services that accompany this type of condition. The family chooses to have the child remain in the home but understands they need assistance because the child's care is around the clock. Financing for this type of care is very expensive and typically not covered under traditional insurance. The case managers work with a home care agency to negotiate rates for 24-hour care and secure needed equipment.

Many catastrophic events result in legal settlements. Once a claim is settled, the court establishes a structured payment system to pay for services, equipment, and other needs the person has as a result of his or her condition.

When private-duty care is needed, a family may elect to hire a team of nurses, which works privately to care for a person who requires private-duty nursing. In this case, the family becomes the employer and is responsible for paying salaries to the individual nurses, for providing benefits, such as workers' compensation and sick time, and for reporting salaries for tax purposes. Many times, an independent case manager or life care planner assists with this type of coordination and should encourage the family to seek expert advice about what their responsibilities are when undertaking this type of project, because it is important to follow the various federal and state requirements that apply to employment.

Subacute Setting

Many times, a patient does not meet the intensity of services necessary for an inpatient acute setting and can receive care in a less-intensive setting in a subacute facility. To ensure appropriate use of resources and to conserve costs, some managed care organizations have implemented processes that allow patients to be admitted directly from an emergency department to a subacute facility if the patient requires more care than can be provided at home but does not meet criteria for acute care.

Case Simulation: An 80-year-old man is admitted to the emergency department (ED) with shortness of breath, sweating, and bilateral pedal edema. The ED physician orders oxygen, a diuretic, and a Foley catheter, as well as lab work, an ECG, arterial blood gases, and a chest x-ray. After a few hours, the physician reevaluates the patient and finds him sitting up, eating a light lunch, and talking with the patient in the next bed. The patient's labs, ABGs, and ECG are within normal limits, but because of the presence of some fluid in the lung and past history of heart disease, the ED physician recommends admission. The patient's managed care organization calls the hospitalist to evaluate the patient, and it is decided that he is stable for transfer to a subacute facility for observation. The patient is agreeable to this, so arrangements are made for the transfer.

Another need that subacute facilities meet is to provide a venue for those who require rehabilitation but do not currently meet the requirements for acute rehabilitation because of their conditions.

Case Simulation: A 68-year-old patient with diabetes has had a stroke and requires rehabilitation services. Because of her overall condition, the patient is not physically able to endure the 3 hours of acute rehabilitation required for admission to the acute rehabilitation facility. Arrangements are made for the patient to be transferred to a subacute setting so she can regain some strength in a less intensive setting. The subacute setting is used as a "bridge" that enables the patient to gain sufficient physical strength to meet the 3-hour rehabilitation requirements of the rehabilitation center.

Skilled Nursing and Long-Term Care

Skilled nursing facilities are centers for patients who have long-term needs and are unable to care for themselves for various reasons. Many of the patients who reside in these centers are elderly, but skilled nursing facilities can also focus on children, adolescents, or adults who have severe disabilities. The goal of these centers is to maintain the maximum health status for the residents and to care for them in a humane and compassionate manner. Family members are encouraged to visit those in skilled care facilities because many times patients cannot advocate for themselves. If abuse is suspected, information should be reported to the state agency that oversees skilled care facilities in the state where the facility is located. Case managers who work in skilled care facilities should ensure that residents are well cared for, and if issues arise, they are addressed proactively. In addition, case managers should ensure that each patient has a current advance directive in place so that if a patient takes a turn for the worse, all understand the patient's wishes regarding emergency care. This information should be communicated to the acute care setting as well, so that care is in line with the patient's wishes.

Custodial Long-Term Care

The focus of long-term care is on specific populations that require professional or personal services on a recurring or continuous basis because of aging or the presence of a chronic or permanent physical or mental impairment. Populations that fall under this category include the elderly, because of their age and inability to function; adults who suffer from chronic illness, catastrophic injuries, or mental impairments that have left them dependent; and children who require long-term care because of devastating injuries, illnesses, congenital defects, or mental impairments.

Case managers who work with the elderly population and address their long-term care needs are known as *geriatric care managers*. The geriatric care manager is called upon many times by the individual patient, the family, or trust officers to assist with coordination of medical care; transportation; and personal issues such as paying bills, shopping, housecleaning, and general upkeep of the home. The geriatric care manager coordinates these services for the patient to ensure that he or she is safe and receiving appropriate services that provide maximum independence. Payment for services provided by the geriatric care manager is usually made on a fee-for-service basis by whoever contracts the service. Adult children of aging parents often contract directly with geriatric care managers. Many companies that specialize in long-term care insurance employ geriatric care managers to assist with care once a policy is activated. Today, many people are planning ahead and purchasing long-term care policies that will be available to them if and when the need arises.

Children with chronic conditions also have special healthcare needs and require frequent use of medical services, equipment, supplies, medications, and access to community resources. Children who fall into this category are children with birth and genetic anomalies, complications from birth that have left them disabled and dependent, and various accidents that have caused permanent damage, such as near-drowning or brain and spinal cord injuries. Case managers who work with this population—either in private practice or through a government agency, such as Medicaid or Children's Medical Services—are most successful when relationships are formed among families, physicians, and nurse care coordinators because the children's needs are so diverse.

Patients over 21 years of age and under the age of 65 with long-term needs often are covered by private health insurance. The payer-based case manager usually addresses the needs of this population if the person has private insurance. Other sources of coverage are found through either Medicaid or Medicare. If the injury or illness resulted from an accident or work-related injury, coverage will be provided by a workers' compensation carrier. If the injury was the result of an accident, a legal settlement may have set up a trust that provides money for long-term care needs or medical care not covered by insurance. In many such cases, a life care plan is done to determine the needs of the person so that structured payments can be arranged to address the future needs of the patient over his or her lifetime. In this event, a trust officer or bank may be responsible for dispensing funds for long-term care. An independent case manager or the workers' compensation case manager may assist with management of care for this population, too. If the case manager is not involved, the family or primary caregiver assumes this role.

As technology continues to improve, allowing people to survive diseases and catastrophic injuries, and our population ages, increased attention is being given to those who require long-term care. As a result of this trend, case managers need to become familiar and comfortable with dealing with the medical, social, and ethical issues that face these populations. A proactive approach to assessment, management of ongoing care needs, and support for those who require long-term care is essential so that problems can be recognized early, treatment initiated, and costs controlled. The goals for case managers who work with these populations are to ensure that each patient reaches his or her maximum potential and to provide education on how to navigate the complex healthcare system effectively and efficiently.

Another aspect of the growing long-term care population is the impact on the caregiver. According to the National Family Caregivers Association (NFCA), more than 65 million people, 29% of the U.S. population, provide care for a chronically ill, disabled, or aged family member or friend during any given year and spend an average of 20 hours per week providing care for their loved one (National Family Caregivers Association, 2009).

The value of the services family caregivers provide for "free," when caring for older adults, is estimated to be **$375 billion** a year. That is almost **twice as much** as is actually spent on homecare and nursing home services combined ($158 billion; National Alliance for Caregiving and Evercare, 2009).

Case managers must take time to educate and inform caregivers about creative ways to deal with challenges that arise from caring for the frail elderly, or people with catastrophic or chronic conditions.

Assisted Living

Assisted living is a venue many seniors are moving toward when they can no longer function in their own homes. An assisted living facility allows a person to live in his or her own apartment or room and then join the community for activities and meals. This type of setting allows the elderly person to remain relatively independent but with some assistance to ensure safety and proper nutrition. Many churches or community agencies have set up assisted living programs for those who are catastrophically ill or disabled because of mental or physical conditions. Safety and proactive management to ensure adherence to treatment are important in this population. Assisted living programs can also provide respite care for families that have elderly or disabled members. These programs allow caregivers to continue to work or have a break from the daily routine while the disabled person is cared for in a safe environment.

Outpatient Treatment Facilities

Other growing resources that case managers refer patients to are infusions and wound care centers. These specialty centers offer specific services for patients. Infusions centers are set up for patients to receive various types of medications in a convenient and comfortable location. Professionals who work at these centers specialize in starting intravenous lines to deliver the medication using the safest and most direct routes. Types of services offered at infusions centers include chemotherapy, various types of pain management treatments, administration of intravenous antibiotics, biologic response modifiers, hydration therapy, blood transfusions, and other therapies that do not require hospitalization.

As a result of the advances in wound care, specialty wound care centers are also now widely available. Nonhealing wounds require specialized services to ensure effective outcomes. Therapies provided by wound care centers include hyperbaric oxygen therapy, whirlpool therapy, nutritional counseling, physical therapy, infection control, and a host of other methods proven to assist the healing process. In addition, wound care centers bring together specialists who consult on wound care management. These specialists include internists, vascular surgeons, general surgeons, plastic and reconstructive surgeons, podiatrists, and nurses and therapists who are certified in wound care management. Working as a team, these specialists evaluate patients and then place them on regimens specific to their individual needs.

Centers also provide professionals and members of the community who may have family members at risk with proactive education on topics such as advances in wound care and prevention.

REIMBURSEMENT SYSTEMS

Healthcare payer systems in the United States are arguably among the most diverse and complex in the world. This section is intended to briefly define the commonalities and differences among reimbursement systems, and to discuss the key points necessary for a case manager to understand when navigating various payer systems. It is not intended to provide current options available in managed care plans, since benefit plans are widely variable and continue to shift to meet the dynamic needs of the healthcare industry. As part of the case management process of assessment, case managers are charged with investigating the benefits that are available to meet the individual needs of the patients they manage. This requires the case manager to have a working knowledge of various reimbursement methods, so as needs arise, options can be analyzed and explored.

Government Reimbursement Systems

Medicare

Medicare is a federally funded government program that was enacted by federal legislation in 1965 and is administered by the Centers for Medicare & Medicaid Services (CMS) within the U.S. Department of Health and Human Services (HHS). Most people age 65 and older are entitled to Medicare Part A, which is considered hospital insurance. Part A covers inpatient hospital services, skilled nursing facilities, approved home health services, and hospice care. Persons eligible for Medicare include those eligible for Social Security Income retirement benefits, for Railroad Retirement benefits, and those under 65 who have been eligible for Social Security Disability Income (SSDI) benefits for at least 24 months (U.S. Department of Health and Human Services, 2011). Examples include persons with a mental impairment, a catastrophic illness, or a chronic illness. Persons may claim Medicare 24 months after the date of injury or after the illness is diagnosed and documented by a physician. There is a 5-month waiting period for persons seeking eligibility. A "fast-track" application process exists for those diagnosed with a terminal illness and who are considered to have 6 months or less to live. Persons under age 65 who have kidney disease that "appears irreversible and permanent and requires a regular course of dialysis or kidney transplantation to maintain life" are also eligible for Medicare Part A (HHS, 2011).

Medicare Part A recipients are automatically eligible for Medicare Part B (medical insurance), providing that they can pay the designated monthly premiums established through insurance companies that provide Part B coverage. Part B covers physician services, outpatient hospital services, and medical equipment and supplies. Premiums for Part B insurance vary widely, particularly because some Part B policies are fee-for-service, or indemnity, plans and some are managed care plans. Senior citizens may have excellent Part B coverage, more limited managed care coverage, or no Part B coverage at all (U.S. Department of Health and Human Services, 2012). Through a managed care plan's "prescription card coverage," they may have some drug benefits and be responsible for a copay on prescription drugs.

> Under the Medicare Prescription Drug, Improvement and Modernization Act (MMA) of 2003, seniors and people living with disabilities were eligible for a voluntary prescription drug benefit effective in 2006. Today this benefit is referred to as the Medicare Prescription Drug Coverage (Part D). Medicare offers prescription drug coverage to everyone with Medicare. The intent of the MMA is to offer more choices and better benefits. In fact, approval of the MMA represented the most significant improvement to senior health care in nearly 40 years. Passage of the MMA was also intended to offer more health plan choices, including regional preferred provider organizations (PPOs), to provide better benefits, higher quality care and substantial cost savings to Medicare beneficiaries. (CMS, 2012c)

In addition to the standard drug benefit, which is available to all beneficiaries with a 75% premium subsidy, passage of the MMA provides low-income seniors and people with disabilities who have limited means—about a third of all people with Medicare—with greater access to coverage, offering limited premiums and deductibles and no coverage gaps. Medicare beneficiaries with retiree coverage benefit from a set of options to obtain more affordable enhanced coverage, including a new retiree drug subsidy, as well as options for employers and unions to wrap around Medicare coverage or offer Medicare-subsidized drug coverage themselves. In addition, states, other persons, and charitable organizations can contribute toward a beneficiary's out-of-pocket costs and still have those contributions count toward catastrophic coverage.

Initially under Medicare Part B, physicians were paid a "usual and customary fee" for particular services. When diagnosis-related groups (DRGs) were unveiled in late 1993, physicians began receiving payments under a resource-based relative value scale (RBRVS) system. Hospitals were paid through the prospective payment system (PPS), which used the DRG process and formulas. DRG payments were based largely upon diagnosis and expected length of stay, so physicians no longer had incentives to keep patients in the hospital. As hospital systems became more astute at collaborating with their physicians for aggressive discharge planning, costs were reduced significantly. In the 1990s, managed care plans assumed the risk of Medicare to target similar cost savings through their managed care Part B plans. Some plans were successful, while others announced "an end" to covering Medicare beneficiaries based on significant losses in managing this often frail population

A Medicare Advantage Plan (like an HMO or PPO) is another Medicare health plan choice patients may have as part of Medicare. Medicare Advantage Plans, sometimes called "Part C" or "MA Plans," are offered by private companies approved by Medicare (CMS, 2012c).

Medicaid

Another fragile population is the Medicaid population, which is served through joint federal and state programs and varies state to state in covered benefits. Medicaid was enacted in 1965 under Title XIX of the Social Security Act. Eligibility for Medicaid is based on income and other financial resources of the applicant. In addition to financial need, an individual may qualify for Medicaid based on medical need as well as categorical need, meaning that the person is already receiving some form of government benefits, such as SSI. If a child is under the age of 21 and has impairment severe enough to meet the disability standards under SSI, the parental income is disregarded in determining Medicaid benefits (CMS, 2012b).

The provision of Medicaid benefits can vary somewhat from state to state, although in all states Medicaid pays for skilled home healthcare nursing services, as well as for long-term care in a nursing home, provided minimum financial requirements are met. Within broad guidelines established by the federal government, each state sets criteria for its Medicaid program, including

- ▶ Eligibility standards;

- ▶ Type, amount, duration, and scope of eligible services;

- ▶ Rate of payment for services offered; and

- ▶ Administration of the program.

Children's Health Insurance

The State Children's Health Insurance Program (SCHIP) is administered by the Centers for Medicare and Medicaid Services and makes funds available to the states that have in place federally approved programs that provide health insurance coverage to uninsured children. The program gives each state permission to offer health insurance for children up to age 19 who are not already insured. SCHIP is a state-administered program and each state sets its own guidelines regarding eligibility and service (CMS, 2012a).

U.S. Department of Veterans Affairs

The U.S. Department of Veterans Affairs (VA) is a part of the military health system that is responsible for providing benefits and health care to our country's men and women who have served in the armed forces. The VA offers vocational and education programs, life insurance, home loans, benefits for dependents and survivors, and death benefits.

Military Health System

The U.S. Military Health Service System (MHSS) uses a managed care delivery system known as TRICARE. TRICARE was initiated to manage the rising costs of health care in the military. It is operated under the Department of Defense and is the nation's largest healthcare system, with more than 8.3 million individuals eligible to receive care. All active duty and retired military personnel and their families, and survivors of active duty military personnel who are not eligible for Medicare based upon age, can participate in one of three levels of TRICARE. Additionally, persons under the age of 65 who are eligible for Medicare because of disability and end-stage renal disease may also choose to participate.

The three levels of TRICARE are TRICARE Prime, TRICARE Standard, and TRICARE Extra. All active duty men and women are automatically enrolled in TRICARE Prime. The focus of TRICARE Prime is to keep the enrollees "fit for duty." In this regard, TRICARE Prime leads the nation in providing a coordinated, systemwide wellness program. TRICARE Prime uses a strong case management and disease management approach to support its wellness program and illness and injury prevention model. Other eligible military personel can choose among the Prime, Standard, and Extra levels of TRICARE. Once retired military personnel, their families, and survivors reach 65, they are eligible for Medicare and are not usually eligible for TRICARE.

TRICARE Standard is the option that provides the most flexibility for TRICARE-eligible beneficiaries. It is a fee-for-service option that gives beneficiaries the opportunity to see any TRICARE-authorized provider. TRICARE Standard is not available to active duty members. Standard shares most of the costs of medically necessary care from civilian providers when care in a military treatment facility is not available.

TRICARE Extra is another option under the MHSS. With TRICARE Extra, beneficiaries do not have to enroll or pay an annual fee, but do have to satisfy an annual deductible for outpatient care. In the TRICARE Extra program, beneficiaries receive discounts on cost sharing and do not have to file their own claims. This option is not available for overseas or active duty service members (TRICARE, 2011).

Private Insurance

Health Maintenance Organizations

A health maintenance organization (HMO) provides health care for people in a specified geographic area. The HMO accepts responsibility for delivering an agreed-to set of services and products to an enrolled group. The HMO collects a predetermined periodic payment in advance (usually on the first of each month) on behalf of each enrollee. Each enrollee is then responsible for assuming a copayment that can vary in cost when seeking the services of a primary care physician (PCP), specialty physician, diagnostic center, or treatment facility. Enrollees are required to seek services from specific providers listed as the HMO's network providers. Enrollees are also required to first seek the medical attention of a preappointed primary care provider (classified as a gatekeeper), rather than independently assuming the need for treatment by a specialty provider. Most specialty providers, with the usual exception of pediatricians, internists, and gynecologists, are covered through the HMO only if the patient sees them based upon a written referral from his or her PCP. The specialist must be an authorized provider in the insurance company's network, or preauthorization for his or her services must have been provided by the insurance company as an out-of-network service.

The primary goal of an HMO is to enhance quality of care through a coordinated network. It is not to enhance cost savings through limitation of benefits—although many still accuse HMOs of rationing health care through limitation of benefits and rewarding gatekeepers for not referring patients for treatment or specialty care. The debates will no doubt continue as HMOs continue to occupy an even larger share of the managed care market.

Preferred Provider Organizations

Preferred provider organizations (PPOs) were designed and implemented as a result of a growing desire by providers to control their own destinies. Providers banded together and formed professional groups, which pool resources and work together to manage the care of patients, referring only to providers who are part of their network. They also have stronger negotiating powers with managed care organizations and other payer groups to provide high-quality care at a reduced cost. Enrollees are encouraged, and sometimes given incentives, to use these preferred providers.

Point-of-Service Provider

There are many options offered in insurance benefit packages. One such option is point-of-service (POS) plans offered by both HMOs and PPOs. This option offers enrollees greater flexibility in choosing providers either in or out of the managed care network for an additional premium cost. There are several types of POS plans offered by insurers. Many are open-access HMOs, whereby the guidelines of an HMO apply but without a confined network of providers from which to choose. There is also what is known as "the gatekeeper model," which may limit access to specialty physicians by requiring a referral from the primary care provider (gatekeeper). Still another type of POS allows open access into and out of the network, but imposes financial penalties for stepping outside the network.

Self-Insured

Today, large companies and employer groups have decided to self-insure for health care instead of purchasing health insurance from a carrier. To do this, an actuary assesses the member population and recommends an amount of money to put into reserve for payment of claims. Traditionally, a third-party administrator (TPA) is engaged to handle the claims administration service for self-funded companies and employer groups. TPAs assume administrative responsibility at a fixed rate to handle all claims; to process claims; to handle all customer correspondence, complaints, appeals, and so forth; and to act as a liaison between the payer and the provider groups. TPAs undertake the heavy paperwork associated with care coordination and documentation systems that self-funded groups are often not equipped or financially able to handle. Many self-insured groups employ TPAs to act as their claims' administration arm. Case managers often report to TPAs because TPAs are responsible for managing those aspects of care coordination that the case manager influences—cost, quality, and access to care.

Forms of Payment

Fee for Service

Fee for service is a method of payment whereby providers are paid for each service performed. An example of fee for service is a provider who does not participate in a managed care arrangement and bills the insurer for each service performed.

Capitation

Capitation is a method of payment under managed care in which healthcare providers are paid a fixed amount for each person over a specific period of time, regardless of the actual number or nature of services and products provided to each person. A fixed monthly payment is provided for each member covered in the plan, regardless of whether the plan member utilizes, underutilizes, or overutilizes the provider's services. This is referred to as *per member, per month*.

Prospective Pay and Diagnostic-Related Groups

The Prospective Pay System was enacted in 1983 and significantly changed Medicare reimbursement from a fee-for-service system to services reimbursed at a predetermined fixed price formulated through diagnostic-related groups.

Diagnostic-related group (DRG) pricing formula was established by Medicare in the mid-1980s. It was modeled to align reimbursement with diagnostic categories. At that time, DRGs were a hot topic and the phrase that became very popular was "patients were being discharged quicker and sicker." The financial implications of the new DRG payment system caused hospitals administrators to reassess their care delivery system—staffing, lengths of stay, policies, procedures, and customer satisfaction. To remain financially viable, hospitals were forced to identify ways to reduce and contain costs by reducing the length of stay, examine the appropriateness of intensity of service, and identify areas of opportunity to improve efficiencies.

Hospital administrators began to look at how the hospital was organized and analyzed the concept of cost centers. The UR department played an important role in this analysis. UR nurses were charged with the responsibility of moving the patient quickly and efficiently through the hospital system and decreasing the length of stay by taking active roles in resource management. They were expected to ensure that any diagnostic tests performed on a Medicare patient were medically necessary. If there was no clear rationale provided in the medical record, the provider who ordered the diagnostic test was consulted regarding its appropriateness. To improve efficiency, if diagnostic tests were not performed in a timely manner, supervisors were held accountable. Furthermore, as soon as diagnostic reports were available in the patient's chart, the UR nurse called the provider to discuss the results and ask for the next step in the treatment plan. This change in patient management created adversarial relationships throughout the entire healthcare system but was justified by administration as a means to remain fiscally viable.

> APDRGs: The All Patient Refined Diagnosis-Related Groups (APR-DRGs) expand the basic DRG structure by adding two sets of subclasses to each base APR-DRG. Each subclass set consists of four subclasses: one addresses patient differences relating to severity of illness and the other addresses differences in risk of mortality. Severity of illness is defined as the extent of physiologic decompensation or organ system loss of function. Risk of mortality is defined as the likelihood of dying. (3M, 2011)

Subrogation

Subrogation refers to the right of an insurance company or self-insured employer to be repaid for the cost of medical care or wage-loss benefits. Repayment is sought from any money a policy holder receives in a lawsuit or any settlement from a third party. There are many instances and many reimbursement systems in which subrogation can occur. An example is seen in the case of a workers' compensation claim. In this instance, the workers' compensation carrier recovered a portion of medical payments and wage losses paid to an injured worker when the injured worker received a settlement from a malpractice case, which concluded that the manufacturer of the equipment that caused the worker's injury was responsible because the equipment was defective.

Stop Loss

The insuring by one insurer for the liability of another insurer when a certain threshold has been met is known as a *stop loss* or *reinsurance*. Thus, reinsurance carriers are also known as *stop-loss carriers*. Reinsurance coverage is common in high-risk claims, such as workers' compensation catastrophic injuries, or some chronic illnesses. The reinsurer works closely with the primary insurance company and requires notification when claims reach a certain threshold. Often the reinsurer requires that case management and utilization management be automatically assigned as or before the threshold is met as part of its stop-loss plan. This is illustrated when a group health insurance company exceeds claims of $200,000 for a plan member. In this example, the company's reinsurance company may assume the risk for any ongoing claims. This doesn't mean that the health insurance company is waived of its responsibility to provide coverage for the member—the member could have benefits that exceed $1 million dollars. What it means is that the health insurance plan's reinsurance company will reimburse claims dollars spent beyond the first $200,000.

Disability Insurance

Disability insurance generally provides periodic payments to replace income lost when an insured person is unable to work as a result of an injury or illness. Typically, disability insurance is packaged under short-term disability (STD) and long-term disability (LTD) policies that may or may not provide medical services along with wage replacement. STD pays benefits during the time a disability exists to a covered person who remains disabled for a specified period, often not to exceed 2 years. LTD insurance is issued to a group or individual and provides a reasonable replacement of a portion of income lost because of a serious or prolonged illness. STD plans can dovetail into LTD plans or stand alone. Likewise, LTD plans can be available without STD benefits.

An important aspect of disability insurance is the "own occ/any occ" rule. Salary replacement can be based upon the plan holder's own occupation (own occ) or any comparable occupation (any occ), depending upon the plan's benefit. Under the "own occ" provision, a person may receive wage loss replacement even if limited from performing only one aspect of an entire job.

Case Simulation: An insurance-based case manager has a chronic back injury that prevents him from driving for an extended period of time. His job as a field case manager requires him to visit hospitals all over the region once a week to review progress of members who are hospitalized. The remainder of the time, the case manager works telephonically from the insurance company's corporate office. The case manager is able to perform all other aspects of his job from his modified workstation in the corporate office, even though he cannot perform the extensive traveling 1 day a week. Since he holds an "own occ" LTD policy, the case manager qualifies for salary replacement benefits, even though he can perform the majority of his work.

Some plans pay only wage losses for the policy holder's own occupation for a specific period of time; thereafter, the wage loss payments can be based upon an "any occ" rate. "Any occ" plans usually have time limitations, often being no less than 1 year, but no more than 5 years. Under an "any occ" provision, the same case manager with the same physical limitation is looked at very differently. Although he cannot perform one aspect of his job, he can perform all tasks required in the company's internal case manager position, which would not require him to leave the office. In this scenario, he may be ineligible for any benefits, or he may receive wage loss benefits based upon the salary of the internal case manager, even if his salary as a field case manager is greater. Further, the disability insurance company's case manager may work with this employee's physician to arrange for a modified job description for the injured case manager, under which he can continue to work without traveling. This would eliminate or reduce the injured case manager's ability to receive salary replacement.

It is important to remember that disability insurance coverage is plan-specific. Although the "own occ/any occ" rule exists, benefit coverage and limitations vary with the policy. Regardless of the type of coverage, the role of the disability insurance case manager is to promote early intervention, high-quality medical care, and customized transitional return-to-work programs, as well as to integrate disability insurance and workers' compensation benefits when available. One of the major differences between disability case management and workers' compensation case management is that the disability case manager generally cannot direct medical care, but can help control costs and outcomes by facilitating a patient's return to work. The disability case manager often requests that the primary care physician evaluate the functional level of the patient to explore the ability of the patient to return to gainful employment, whether at the existing job, a modified version of the job, or a different job.

Workers' Compensation

Workers' compensation is a no-fault, individually state–governed insurance system that addresses work-related injuries and illnesses. Since 1911, when the Workers' Compensation Act was enacted (see Chapter 5), states have been mandated through employer-sponsored programs to govern wage replacement and medical benefits for both temporary and permanent disabilities, regardless of whether the employer or the worker is at fault for the injury or illness. The goal of workers' compensation is to provide prompt medical care coordination to return the worker to gainful reemployment. More information on workers' compensation is covered in Chapter 5.

Vocational Rehabilitation

Vocational rehabilitation (VR) is provided with eligibility criteria set by individual states in accordance with federal law. In general, to be eligible for services provided through state VR programs, persons must have a physical or mental impairment that impedes employment, and must be reasonably expected to become employable as a result of services provided. In this regard, a disabled child who is not nearing the employment age of 16 is not eligible for VR services. Likewise, a disabled individual over the retirement age of 70 is not eligible. The intent is to address the individual's physical, mental, behavioral, and environmental needs so that successful, gainful employment can be achieved, moving the disabled person to self-reliance and independence.

VR is often termed "the payer of last resort." In addition to funding medical services, it provides training and education for persons who otherwise have little or no medical or vocational coverage. Services provided include

▶ Vocational training,

▶ Higher education necessary to achieve appropriate employment (e.g., an associate's degree from a school of nursing or a bachelor's degree in computer technology),

▶ Financial support during rehabilitation,

▶ Communication services (e.g., readers and note-takers to assist a blind candidate while in a school or training institution funded by VR), and

▶ Physical and mental rehabilitation services (e.g., acute and postacute medical care; prosthetic and assistive devices; transportation; home and jobsite modifications for independence; therapies, such as occupational, physical, and speech therapy).

SUPPORT SERVICES

Emergency Services

Assisting patients with locating emergency and essential services is an key aspect of resource management. Today, there are a wealth of local, state, and federal resources to assist those in need of emergency housing, clothing, or food. Local police, emergency assistance offices, disaster relief services, and others offer a host of resources that can be tapped into as needed. An example of a 24-hour, 7-day-a-week national service is 2-1-1. This service was developed by the United Way, with funding through the federal government, and offers referral services, crisis management, and critical services to meet the needs of people in need (United Way, 2012). Case managers can use this toll-free number or online resource to locate a range of needed services or can provide the number to patients. Another resource for locating housing for the elderly is SNAP for Seniors. SNAP (www.snapforseniors.com) provides a free, online service that allows users to search for senior housing information using tools designed to match the person's needs and care level. A third source that many case managers find useful is the *Case Management Resource Guide* (published by Dorland Health). This is a trusted resource for case managers to locate a wide variety of resources, such as social service agencies, equipment, and a multitude of other products and services. In addition to the hard-copy version of the guide, there is a free online version available at www.cmrg.com.

Collaboration with social workers is important when challenged with securing resources to address patient's nonmedical needs. These experts help people cope with the many safety and quality issues that can arise throughout the course of their everyday lives by directing patients and family members to appropriate services to meet their needs.

Volunteer Organizations

Community resources are a fundamental component of resource management, and volunteer organizations are a fundamental component of community resources. Case managers wishing to ensure successful resource management must have a reliable list of voluntary organizations in their community. Finding volunteer organizations and pertinent contact information is achieved by talking to local church groups, civic organizations, and the chamber of commerce. Case managers will find that each community has a variety of resources once they begin to search.

National support groups also are important resources and can be tapped into for those with major illnesses and injuries. A few examples include the American Heart Association, the Brain Injury Association of America, and the National Hospice Foundation. These support groups are accessible via the Internet, national toll-free numbers, and local chapters. Major nonprofit organizations, such as the Red Cross and the United Way, provide extensive lists of smaller volunteer organizations available in local areas. These are usually printed in educational pamphlets intended for consumers. Hospital emergency departments traditionally keep similar lists as resources for patients and may include support groups germane to the hospital system that are not otherwise listed in consumer resource pamphlets. Religious organizations are excellent sources of such lists, too, and include interdenominational organizations that may not be found on other resource lists. Of course, there's also the Internet, a valuable tool that professionals, as well as patients, can use to search for resources.

Social Services

Social service agencies are excellent resources for patients who require assistance with food stamps, financial counseling, and so on, and for those adults and children who have special needs. Most social service organizations usually require that the patient meet certain eligibility criteria not required by volunteer organizations. Social service agencies are financed by county, state, and federally matched funds and, therefore, are not usually as flexible or timely in meeting individual needs. However, social service agencies provide more intense services over longer periods of time than do voluntary services.

Examples of social service agencies that can help case managers obtain community resources for patients are centers for independent living (CIL), area state-run vocational rehabilitation offices, local departments of social services (LDSS), and local Area Agency on Aging offices. Case managers should maintain logistical information on area social service agencies, including basic eligibility criteria; office(s) where applications for assistance can be made; the qualifying waiting period, if any; and other pertinent information. Some case managers request and keep a supply of eligibility forms for potential patients' use.

Case Simulation: *A case manager covering the obstetrics unit of a hospital has Women, Infants and Children (WIC) program information on hand to assist a financially insecure new mother obtain free formula for her newborn.*

Public Health Services

Public health agencies provide broad services, such as vaccinations to protect against diseases; screenings for lead poisoning and tuberculosis; testing to ensure the safety of food, water, and drugs; investigations to control the outbreak of infectious disease; collection of health statistics to develop prevention and regulatory programs; screening of newborns for genetic diseases; and programs to meet the special needs of women (Illinois Department of Public Health, 2008).

Another aspect of public health services is public health clinics, which are found in most communities and provide important services. Primary care providers and nurse practitioners are available to provide community-sensitive services that are free or are offered on a sliding payment scale to anyone walking through their doors. Primary health care typically includes medical and dental care, mental health services, well-child immunizations, adult inoculations to prevent community-acquired diseases (e.g., influenza, pneumonia), and birth control products and services. Community outreach classes are usually offered on a continuing basis and provide information about smoking cessation, weight loss, the dangers of drug use and abuse, domestic violence, and communicable diseases.

Part of the public health services' role in protecting public health is being aware of communicable diseases. Therefore, each state's public health department requires that first responders and healthcare professionals report certain communicable diseases in an effort to reduce the risk to public health. Such reporting allows public health professionals to investigate the claim, and set processes in place to contain and limit exposure. Examples of reportable events include anthrax exposure, sexually transmitted infections, hepatitis, tuberculosis, HIV infection, meningitis, animal bites, and persons who are dead on arrival (DOA). Healthcare professionals should be familiar with the reportable events and procedures for reporting because they vary from state to state. Documentation of all reports made is an essential part of the process to ensure compliance with state laws.

Educational Services

In order to ensure that children with catastrophic injuries or chronic medical conditions have access to education, a federal act—the Education for All Handicapped Children Act—was passed in 1975. This legislation

▶ Provides the right for all disabled children to receive "free appropriate public education";

▶ Promotes equal educational opportunities, despite a child's degree of disability or the services needed to achieve equality;

▶ Establishes procedures by which disabled children are evaluated and classified; and

▶ Provides for the development and implementation of appropriate programs of special education and "related services" stemming from the evaluations and classifications. These individualized education programs (IEPs) are developed jointly by school officials and parents (New York City Department of Education, 2012).

Early intervention programs provide services for children less than 5 years of age. These services usually include physical, occupational, and speech therapies.

Case Simulation: *An 8-year-old child who survived a near-drowning accident is discharged home following extensive rehabilitation. The case manager contacts the local school system to discuss the services available for the child. A family meeting is set up with a representative from the school system, the parents, and the case manager. The school system representative informs all about the resources the school system provides to meet the child's needs. The parents are invited to visit one of the schools in their community that provides education to medically complex children. In addition, a nurse is on staff to handle the medical needs of the children. Transportation to and from home also is available. The family is appreciative and feels that having access to these services allows them some normalcy in their lives despite their child's extensive ongoing medical issues.*

Vocational Services

An important role that case managers play, regardless of setting, is assisting patients in obtaining a level of physical and mental wellness that allows them to reach their maximum potential. Depending on the patient's age, this allows people to secure gainful employment within their functional capacities, or, as previously discussed, return to school. Patients who have a catastrophic injury or illness that jeopardizes their ability to work may benefit from vocational services.

To meet this need, case managers collaborate with other members of the healthcare team, the vocational specialists. The vocational specialist has specific education and training that allows him or her to work with patients who have physical and mental challenges. Vocational specialists meet with patients to gain insight into their medical conditions, current work status, level of education, and other aspects of their lives that could have an impact on their ability to work. Following this, the specialist may perform a vocational assessment. Vocational assessments are commonly used in the workers' compensation arena as part of the rehabilitation process, but they can also be used outside of this system as needed.

A *vocational assessment* is a comprehensive process conducted over a period of time to identify the individual characteristics, skills, education, job training, and job placement needs of an ill or injured person. The assessment usually involves a multidisciplinary team that assesses the various aspects required to evaluate the patient's current status. The vocational specialist assesses the patient's work environment to evaluate and understand the current work setting and the skills needed to perform the job. Another aspect of the assessment is a series of tests that evaluate and determine employability. These include

- ▶ Achievement tests (e.g., reading comprehension tests),

- ▶ Aptitude tests (e.g., motor coordination tests),

- ▶ Vocational tests (e.g., ability to make correct choices to supervise others),

- ▶ Work samples (e.g., testing both the ability to weld and the knowledge of welding),

- ▶ Behavioral observation (e.g., observing patient's ability to follow directions during test-taking),

- ▶ Situational assessment (e.g., observing patient's behavior in a simulated or role-playing work setting), and

- ▶ Work observations (e.g., observing the patient in the actual work setting).

Another function of the assessment is to determine the patient's transferable skills. Transferable skills analysis is appropriate when the person's actual or projected physical abilities are too limited to go back to his or her original job. To determine transferable skills, the vocational specialist discusses with the patient his or her work history, education, and training. An analysis is then conducted to profile the past jobs, determining the highest level of vocational functioning. These functions are classified as transferable skills because they are skills that the person can use, or transfer, from one job to another. Transferable skills are based on the result of the person's aptitudes, skills, and physical abilities, and assist the vocational specialist in better understanding the talents of the individual.

A labor-market survey or analysis is often performed when an ill or injured person requires retraining. This analysis searches the local job market to determine job availability for positions suited to the patient's skills, abilities, and physical limitations. The survey, combined with information from the skills analysis, is used for

- ▶ A job search,

- ▶ Career counseling,

- ▶ The study of employment trends, and

- ▶ A wage-loss analysis.

The steps a vocational specialist takes in completing a labor-market survey include determining the focus of the study, identifying the data-gathering method, and determining the final form of the data. In the past decade, Internet access has changed data-gathering methods. Today, vocational specialists are able to perform quick, efficient job searches. Resources used include job search engines, local and national newspapers, and networking with employers through community events (Kuhn & Skuterud, 2000).

Legal Services

Patients have many rights promoted by ethical practice and promulgated by legislation. Patient rights are protected under such well-known healthcare legislative acts as the Patient's Bill of Rights; Health Insurance Portability and Accountability Act (HIPAA), which most recently released mandates to protect patient confidentiality; the Patient Self-Determination Act (PSDA), promoting a patient's right to accept or refuse treatment should he or she become gravely ill or injured; and the Emergency Medical Treatment and Active Labor Act (EMTALA), protecting patients from being refused emergency medical treatment. These laws are discussed in more depth in Chapter 5.

SUPPLIES AND EQUIPMENT

Among the ongoing, often expensive resources required by chronically ill or injured patients are the needs for medical equipment and supplies. Medical equipment and supplies, including durable medical equipment (DME), are available from vendors, home medical equipment companies, home healthcare agencies, and retail pharmacies. Other providers that may sell or provide supplies and equipment include social service and volunteer organizations, hospital therapy and outpatient departments, long-term-care and nursing home facilities, and consignment shops specializing in secondhand equipment. Home medical equipment and supplies are broadly classified into the following product groups:

▶ Ambulation aids, such as walkers, canes, and crutches

▶ Bathing and toileting aids, such as shower chairs, tub lifts, handheld showers, raised toilet seats, and grab bars

▶ Respiratory equipment, such as oxygen concentrators, cannulas, masks, nebulizers, peak flow monitors, and pulse oximeters

▶ Beds, such as manually adjusted or electric beds, mattresses, and trapeze bars

▶ Physical therapy equipment, such as treadmills, stationary bikes, weights, Transcutaneous Electrical Nerve Stimulator (TENS) units, and continuous passive motion machines

▶ Wound care equipment, such as low air loss mattresses and wound care dressings

▶ Enteral products, such as nutrition pumps, tube feeding and oral nutritional supplements, and gastrostomy feeding tubes

▶ Wheelchairs and accessories, such as manual and power wheelchairs, seat cushions, and storage compartments

▶ Personal assistive products, such as reachers, glucose-monitoring devices, blood pressure monitors, and portable ramps

When ordering medical equipment or supplies for a patient, the case manager should follow up to ensure that the equipment is delivered in good working order, and the patient and caregiver are comfortable operating the equipment or using the supplies. Additional training may be required to ensure the patient's safety and health, and to prevent an unnecessary hospital readmission.

The patient and family or caregiver should have information about the equipment agreement that accompanies each piece of equipment. This information includes how the equipment is to be maintained and the responsibility of the user to maintain the equipment. The patient and family or caregiver are provided with contact information from the equipment manufacturer and from the agency or company providing the equipment, in case of equipment failure or if maintenance is required.

Disposables

Another category in the case manager's toolbox is disposables. Disposables include a wide array of products for perineal care and skin care, such as ostomy supplies, wound care supplies (e.g., gauze, bandages, adhesive tape), syringes for insulin, and protective wear for incontinence. Because the use of these products can be lifelong, the case manager carefully compares prices of disposables and uses his or her negotiating skills to create the best agreement that provides high-quality products, on-time delivery, and patient comfort.

Pharmaceuticals

A changing paradigm is pharmaceutical companies providing direct-to-consumer education regarding medication compliance and adherence. Only in recent years have pharmaceutical companies engaged in teaching consumer awareness of drug choice to the general public. Television and print advertising, billboards, and radio announcements are among the mediums used by pharmaceutical companies to deliver their messages to the public. Sophisticated educational Web sites specifically geared toward consumers are also offered by most pharmaceutical companies. In addition, pharmaceutical companies are known to spend thousands of dollars developing consumer education support documents. Available support tools and materials include patient diaries that encourage patients to write questions for future physician visits; care pathways that give patients specific instructions on important nutritional, exercise, functional, and psychosocial interventions for a healthy lifestyle; and a myriad of other educationally based support materials, such as user-friendly videos, pamphlets, audiotapes, checklists, books, magazines, and index cards. These educational efforts are part of a drug-state-management initiative undertaken by pharmaceutical companies that believe that educated consumers will advocate for and demand certain drugs from their primary care and specialist providers.

Case managers can tap into many of these consumer education materials produced by pharmaceutical firms for their personal professional use, or to help patients, families, and caregivers better understand this messaging. Often, case managers can access this wealth of educational tools by logging on to various pharmaceutical companies' Web sites and selecting either consumer or healthcare professional portals. Many pharmaceutical companies exhibit at national and regional case management conferences as well. There they display healthcare and consumer educational tools. Another service provided by many pharmaceutical companies is toll-free consumer support lines. Case managers can use these lines to inquire about available educational materials or to access a wide range of resources that serve as professional development tools because they help case managers stay current with available drug therapies, potential comorbid conditions, drug side effects, and symptom management.

Some pharmaceutical companies also provide patient assistance programs for those patients who cannot afford the prescribed drug therapy. Established criteria that explain what patients must do to meet eligibility requirements are also accessible.

The challenge for case managers when using pharmaceutical resources and services is to remain objective. Case managers should also caution patients and family members to objectively view media advertising and educational pieces regarding prescription and over-the-counter medications. Not every drug is right for every patient. Case managers should encourage their patients to speak directly with their physicians regarding available drug options and other treatments, and to ensure that whatever is recommended is based on sound clinical evidence.

Durable Medical Equipment

Durable medical equipment (DME) companies are organizations that provide equipment and other supplies necessary for home medical care. Many DME companies are "one-stop-shops" that case managers can use to order supplies and medications, coordinate nursing care, and arrange for patient transportation. Prior to coordinating services, the case manager or discharge planner should determine whether the patient has insurance or, if not, how to pay for the DME's services or products. Community resources might be an option for patients and family members who cannot afford the equipment or service. For those requiring education, the DME provider or a specialist or consultant can instruct patients and family members on how to use any equipment or supplies that are delivered.

Case Simulation: A patient discharged with end-stage cardiomyopathy requires oxygen for home use. A technician trained by the DME company delivers the oxygen to the patient's home, sets it up, and instructs the patient and his family on how to use and care for the equipment, and on safety issues regarding home oxygen use. The technician asks the patient and family members if they have any questions and leaves a number with them so that if questions come up, they can call for assistance. This type of DME company service provides a sense of security for the patient and his family.

Provider Services

Nurse case managers must have a working knowledge of the provider network, including the following:

▶ Types of providers: MDs, NPs, PA, CNM, etc.

▶ Providers' specialties: cardiology, neurology, OB, endocronology, ENT, etc.

▶ Scope of providers' practices

▶ Location of providers and accessibility

▶ How to access services of out-of-network providers for your patients

▶ Cost of services, including what types of insurance a provider accepts and whether they balance bill patients

As you can clearly see, resource management is a skill that requires honing. Every day in every way, case managers must understand what they need to do and how they need to do it to ensure their patients receive high-quality, effective, and cost-effective care. They must advocate for their patients to ensure that that they receive the right service, at the right time, in the right setting, delivered by the right provider for the right cost. Not an easy task but one a proficient case manager can handle.

REFERENCES

Bower, K., & Falk, C. (1996). Case management as a response to quality, cost, and access imperatives. In E. Cohen (Ed.), *Nurse case management in the 21st century* (pp. 161–167). St. Louis, MO: Mosby.

Carneal, G. (2000). The evolution of utilization management. *Managed Care Interface, 24*(12), 86–92.

Centers for Medicare and Medicaid Services. (2012a). *Children's health plan.* Retrieved from http://www.medicaid.gov/Medicaid-CHIP-Program-Information/Medicaid-and-CHIP-Program-Information.html

Centers for Medicare and Medicaid Services. (2012b). *General information on Medicaid: Keeping America healthy.* Retrieved from http://www.cms.hhs.gov/MedicaidGenInfo

Centers for Medicare and Medicaid Services. (2012c). *Medicare.Gov.* Retrieved from http://www.medicare.gov/navigation/medicare-basics/medicare-benefits/part-c.aspx

Centers for Medicare and Medicaid Services. (2012). *Medicare program–General information.* Retrieved from www.cms.gov/Medicare/Medicare-General-Information/MedicareGenInfo.index.html

Dorland Health. (2012). *Case management resource guide.* Retrieved from www.cmrg.com

Illinois Department of Public Health. (2008). *About the Department.* Retrieved from http://www.idph.state.il.us/about/abouthome.htm

Kuhn, P., & Skuterud, M. (2000). *Job search methods: Internet versus traditional.* Washington, DC: U.S. Government Printing Office.

McKesson, (2012). *Inter Qual decision support.* Retrieved from http://www.mckesson.com/en_us/McKesson.com/Our%2BBusinesses/McKesson%2BHealth%2BSolutions/Solution%2BAreas/InterQual%2BDecision%2BSupport/InterQual%2BDecision%2BSupport.html

Mcleod, S. (2007). *Maslow Hierarchy of Needs.* Retrieved from http://www.simplypsychology.org/maslow.html accessed 02182012

Milliman, (2012). *Milliman care guidelines.* Retrieved from http://www.milliman.com/expertise/healthcare/products-tools/milliman-care-guidelines/

National Alliance for Caregiving and Evercare. *(2009). Evercare survey of the economic downturn and its impact on family caregiving.* Retrieved from http://www.nfcacares.org/who_are_family_caregivers/care_giving_statstics.cfm

National Family Caregivers Association. (2009). *National Family Caregivers national report 2009 fiscal year.* Retrieved from http://www.thefamilycaregiver.org/pdfs/AnnualReport2009.pdf

National Transitions of Care Coalition. (2011). *Home page.* Retrieved from http://www.ntocc.org/Home/tabid/36/Home/tabid/36/Default.aspx

New York City Department of Education. (2012). *Individualized education program.* Retrieved from http://schools.nyc.gov/Offices/District75/Departments/IEP/default.htm

3M. (2011). *AP DRG Classification System.* Retrieved from http://solutions.3m.com/wps/portal/3M/en_US/3M_Health_Information_Systems/HIS/Products/APRDRG/

TRICARE. (2011). *Overview of Tricare benefits.* Retrieved from http://www.military.com/benefits/tricare

U.S. Department of Health and Human Services. (2008). *Medicare hospital prospective payment system. How DRG rates are calculated and updated.* Retrieved from http://oig.hhs.gov/oei/reports/oei-09-00-00200.pdf3

U.S. Department of Health and Human Services. (2010). *Medicare appeals procedures*. Retrieved from http://www.hhs.gov/dab/divisions/medicareoperations/medicare_appeals-procedures.html

U.S. Department for Health and Human Services. (2012). *Office of Consumer Information and Insurance Oversight national health expenditure data*. Retrieved from http://cciio.cms.gov

United Way. (2012). *2-1-1*. Retrieved from http://www.211.org

CHAPTER 4

QUALITY MANAGEMENT

> **"It is easier to do a job right than to explain why you didn't."**
> —*Martin Van Buren*

> **"Quality is never an accident; it is always the result of high intention, sincere effort, intelligent direction and skillful execution; it represents the wise choice of many alternatives."**
> —*William A. Foster*

The field of quality management continues to flourish among all industries in our country, and health care is no exception. Quality planning is being incorporated into all aspects of patient care, and it behooves the nurse case manager to understand the different components of a quality management plan. It is also important to know that a quality management plan focuses on customer satisfaction, prevention of errors, management responsibility, and continuous improvement.

Nurse case managers who serve as project managers should assume responsibility for the development of quality policies for the project and the coordination of related activities, in compliance with any organizational standards, regulatory standards, or both. A quality management plan documents this information and describes the authorities, policies, tools, and techniques that are specific to ensuring project excellence; reducing costs; and eliminating unnecessary corrections, changes, or both. It is developed in the planning phase of a project and focuses on the processes used to plan, implement, document, and asses the project's level of quality. The plan defines the project's policies, objectives, principles, responsibilities, and accountability as it relates to project quality and outlines how the project team will implement, perform, and measure those policies.

It is important to note that the concept of quality does not necessarily require perfection. Quality is more about doing what was agreed to than being perfect or even exceeding expectations.

QUALITY METRICS AND MEASURES

Quality metrics are parameters or ways of quantitatively assessing a project's level of quality, along with the processes to carry out such measurement. Metrics outline the standard that work will be measured against and are often unique to each project or product. Quality metrics are defined in the planning phase of the project and then measured throughout the project's life to track and assess the project's level of conformity to its established quality baseline.

When identifying metrics by which to measure project quality against, an established standard is identified and then used to establish a quality baseline for each defined quality metric. This baseline is then used to measure overall project quality throughout the project's life. Sources of quality baseline information include: the organization's quality plan, similar projects completed within the last 6 months, industry standards, and benchmarks.

When you see the words "quality management," it brings to mind many terms: quality assurance (QA), quality improvement (QI), total quality management (TQM), continuous quality improvement (CQI), and performance improvement (PI). One or another of these terms has been used to describe quality improvement concepts and processes in the healthcare arena since the mid-1980s. Each describes how to measure quality, evaluate compliance, and manage the care and services received by patients and provided by practitioners in all disciplines. These processes contain strategies to assist performance-improvement staff as they examine the quality of health care across professional disciplines and provide feedback for

- ▶ Improving healthcare system performance,
- ▶ Integrating the information derived from all discipline-specific performance-improvement activities, and
- ▶ Ensuring that the information is translated into resource requirements in the planning process.

The discipline of nursing is no exception. Nurse case managers work diligently to make their footprints in the sands of quality management as well. In doing so, they realize that the tools developed to assist them in quality management are data-driven.

Nurse case managers are constantly making decisions on which actions or interventions should be taken in order for some issue to be resolved or a care plan to be developed that will deliver high-quality, cost-effective care and the desired outcomes. They need comparative data to design improvement programs and compare their performances against regional and national benchmarks. Case managers and providers in every discipline are continuously looking for ways to improve the quality of the services they deliver. As the cost of health care continues to rise, the healthcare industry searches for ways to not only maintain quality, but also improve it. Advances in the science of quality measurement, in health information systems, and in the understanding of how to effect change in clinical practice present unprecedented opportunities for improvement. Essential to this is having the right tools to use and the right processes in place to guide you. Quality measurement and reporting are powerful mechanisms that contain both tools and processes to drive quality improvement.

Many of these quality management processes exist and are employed today in case management departments, healthcare facilities, and organizations around the world. Most of these processes utilize tools—some purchased, some built in-house. Regardless of which tools are used, nurse case managers must have input and buy-in from the entire team. It is important that the team understand that the tools are not meant to replace clinical judgment, but are used to guide and organize treatment decisions in specific situations. This chapter will discuss the various aspects of the quality management process and some of the tools popular in today's healthcare systems.

VARIANCE TRACKING

Variances are deviations or variations from a standard or norm. In case management, they are deviations from the recommended interventions in any plan of care or an activity set out in a clinical pathway. Variances can be positive or negative, are the one element unique and essential to all care plans, are recorded by the case manager during the course of care, and allow the case manager to review and update the process of care delivery with attention to patient and other outcomes. As the case manager looks at quality management processes, variance tracking helps identify opportunities for improvement.

Care and case management plans have emerged as the most desirable tools for improving patient care quality through the elimination or prevention of variances, reduction in duplication and fragmentation of care elements, and the standardization of patient care activities. When care and case management plans are followed appropriately, they result in consistency in the practice patterns of physicians, nurses, and other healthcare professionals and, thus, reduce variations in patient care.

To determine care plan variances, the case manager needs to put a stake in the ground as her or his starting point: this is the baseline. Without this, you are chasing and attempting to control a moving target. Two key baselines to establish before you can put variance tracking and reporting into play are cost and time frame. Before you can get there, however, you'll want to work with the patient to establish mutually agreed-upon goals.

In creating a case management plan, case managers must identify a best practice, implement it, track variances, review data, review the contents of the care plan, redraft the plan, and take action to improve care.

Case management professionals use variance tracking as a way to reduce or manage negative occurrences related to the care provided to patients. Variance tracking can also identify positive occurrences that may then be recognized as a standard of care to enhance practice. Variances can occur at any time throughout the course of treatment. They occur when the patient does not progress as outlined according to the clinical pathway and are usually classified according to who or what caused the variance. Variances can be caused by the patient, the individual clinical or healthcare professionals, or because of a fault in the system. When variances to the clinical pathway occur, documentation should note this and what was done to correct the variance at the time. If variances are a result of complex causes, an interdisciplinary case consultation is convened to discuss the events. The meeting focuses on determining whether the pathway is realistic for the individual patient, as well as whether the variance can be resolved. As said previously, variances can occur for several reasons. This next case simulation demonstrates several reasons for negative variances.

Case Simulation: Mr. B. is a 30-year-old Hispanic male admitted by a gastroenterologist, to whom he was referred by his primary care provider, for abdominal pain.

▶ **Patient variance** occurs when a patient's reaction to a procedure or treatment results in complications. *Mr. B. is scheduled for a colonoscopy on Monday. He is instructed to take the required pretest solutions in preparation for the exam. When the patient arrives at the ambulatory care site, he informs the nurse that he was unable to complete the pretest course of solutions, stating he could not swallow all of the solution that was required. Since it will probably be the case that the patient's bowels have not been sufficiently cleaned out for the doctor to perform the exam, the exam is canceled and rescheduled for another date, and there is a consultation about what alternative methods can be used for the cleansing of the bowel and colon.*

▶ **Clinician variance** is any untoward occurrence related to the clinician or professional charged with caring for a patient. *The doctor is unavailable to consult with Mr. B. or the nurse at this time about an alternative preparation for the colonoscopy. Therefore, the patient is asked to call back the next day, and the nurse will have spoken with the doctor by then and will inform the patient of next steps. This delay will cause a delay in diagnosis.*

▶ **System variance** occurs when there is a breakdown related to the healthcare system in general. *The urologist orders a colonoscopy for Mr. B. on a Monday morning but is informed when he arrives that there had been a mistake in the scheduling and that there were two patients scheduled for the same time. The other patient had come in early and was already being prepped for the procedure. The patient is asked to come back on Wednesday. The system is responsible for the variance that will cause the patient inconvenience and some additional discomfort and make it necessary to call to receive a new authorization from the insurance compan for the procedure.*

These examples are very real to case managers in their roles as patient advocates and system navigators. Their goal is to help eliminate or reduce these types of negative variances.

Variance tracking allows an organization to identify areas where problems are occurring and critically evaluate whether changes need to be made. In the examples above, if the variance is impacting the safety of the patient or adversely impacting reimbursement, making changes to correct the variance can be a recommendation by the case manager. Documentation regarding how the variance occurred, along with supporting information on associated costs, provides objective data that can be used to support the need for change.

CONTINUOUS QUALITY IMPROVEMENT (CQI)

Continuous quality improvement is a process in which an attempt is made to optimize the quality output of a system under consideration. Health care in the United States is one such system. Many steps are being taken by several stakeholders—the government, private industry, the military, providers, payers, and consumers—to eliminate waste and non–value-added activities associated with this system. A good CQI process can help make that happen. Even though at times it may seem that quality cannot be defined, case managers still know what quality is; they need to realize that CQI is an unending journey.

A major figure in the quality improvement movement was William Edwards Deming (1900–1993), an American statistician, college professor, author, lecturer, and consultant. Deming is widely credited with improving production in the United States during World War II, although he is perhaps best known for his work in Japan. There, from 1950 onward, he taught top management how to improve design (and thus service), product quality, testing, and sales (the last through global markets), through various methods, including the application of statistical methods such as analysis of variance (ANOVA) and hypothesis testing. Deming made a significant contribution to Japan's later renown for innovative high-quality products and its economic power. He is regarded as having had more impact upon Japanese manufacturing and business than any other individual not of Japanese heritage. Despite being considered something of a hero in Japan, he was only beginning to win widespread recognition in the United States at the time of his death (Paton, 1993). Deming introduced many tools and principles to the process. These are discussed here.

It is important that nurse case managers understand that in order to achieve a stated goal in the CQI process, many things must be considered. Is there an aim? Is there enough time to achieve the aim? Is there a CQI champion? Is there buy-in from the team members and administration? Are there good working relationships among all the players or do they need to be developed?

Because case managers are the professionals who interact with all of the healthcare team members and are often referred to as the "movers and shakers" or "the glue" that holds the system together, it is important that they understand the concepts of quality improvement and the tools needed to engage in the process. One such tool is the Plan-Do-Study-Act, or PDSA, cycle (see Figure 4–1).

Note that PDSA, based on Shewhart's agricultural model of 1939—"Specifications-Production-Inspection"—was refined in 1986 into PDSA. It was then promoted by Deming in his work known as the Plan-Do-Check-Act, or PDCA, cycle. Today, any one of these references will suffice: PDSA, PDCA, Deming Cycle, or Shewhart Cycle. For our purposes, we will refer to it as PDSA.

FIGURE 4–1.
THE PLAN-DO-STUDY-ACT CYCLE

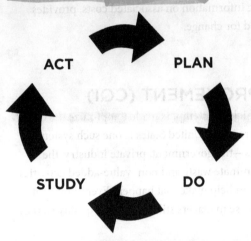

The *PDSA cycle* is a cyclical, four-stage improvement process: Plan-Do-Study-Act. The process promotes continuous quality improvement and includes gathering data on the current situation and history. The "Do" stage is actually an experiment stage, where possible improvements are tested as pilots (on a small scale). During the "Study" stage, the results of those experiments are analyzed. The "Act" stage is used to adopt improvements if the experiment finds successful methods.

All sorts of variations on this improvement process are used. In some models, if more experiments are needed, they are undertaken during the Act stage. Finally, the "Plan" stage is a study of those results and then planning for new experiments. An important practice is to document what improvements are expected during this stage. Failure to document anticipated improvements makes it difficult to learn, and results in the study phase are often neglected altogether. Although key to the success of PDSA is to use it as a cyclical process, often it is not. Instead, the only action is to decide on a modification and do it.

Case Simulation: A nurse case manager identified a need to increase the number of members enrolled in a clinic-sponsored smoking cessation program. The program was funded by one of the organization's contracted health plans. The case manager had read about the PDSA cycle, thought it was interesting and wanted to try it, but first she had to sell the idea to the "powers that be." She researched the issue and presented a plan to administration. The plan was clear, concise, and had a positive return on investment (ROI). The plan named her as the project champion and listed several other members of the team as volunteers to work with her. She described the different strategies she wished to employ and the timeline for implementation, and received the go-ahead from administration.

Her first of many strategies was to give providers a preprinted prescription pad for ordering smoking cessation services for patients, thereby utilizing the provider's face-to-face time with the patient to encourage enrollment in the program and making it easier for the provider to promote the program.

Plan. *Her objective was to increase the number of enrollees (identified smokers) in the smoking cessation program by 10%. Her strategy was to use preprinted prescription pads to increase the number of members enrolled in the smoking cessation program.*

Do. *To implement her strategy, the case manager and a colleague designed the form, had it printed and distributed to the providers working in the clinic, and began to collect data.*

Study. *After 3 months, she noticed no change in the percentage of members enrolled in the program. She set out to learn why not; what went wrong. She learned that the providers were not using the prescription pads. When she asked why, the providers said that when they were seeing the patient they were not aware of what, if any, insurance they have. Therefore, because they could not give every identified patient who smokes the prescription, they gave it to no one. The case manager analyzed this reasoning and agreed that the strategy was far from ideal. She also learned that if she had involved some of the providers in the process from the beginning, she would have learned about this barrier earlier and would not have rolled out the pilot project in this way. She took her lessons learned and spoke to administration about altering her strategy.*

Act. *The case manager received approval to contract with the Department of Health Smokers' Quit Line. Together they enrolled the clinics' patients in the state quit-smoking program. The quit line staff notified the sponsoring health plan about any members who enrolled for the quit line and were then referred to the plan's smoking cessation program. The forms were reprinted with provider input and were in providers' hands within 6 weeks. The program's objective remained the same, only the strategy changed. Three months later, a 2% increase in enrollment was evidenced by the data collected. The plan was working.*

The idea behind the PDSA piece of the CQI process is to take baby steps and evaluate effectiveness sooner and make changes more quickly.

Six Sigma, another quality management process, is a disciplined, data-driven approach and methodology for eliminating defects in any process—from manufacturing to transactional sale or movement of product from product to service. Some healthcare organizations subscribe to this approach for the quality management process.

Six Sigma describes quantitatively how a process is performing, driving toward six standard deviations between the mean and the nearest specification limit. To achieve Six Sigma, a process must not produce more than 3.4 defects per million opportunities. A Six Sigma defect is defined as anything outside of customer specifications.

The fundamental objective of the Six Sigma methodology is the implementation of a measurement-based strategy that focuses on process improvement and variation reduction through the use of two Six Sigma submethodologies: DMAIC and DMADV. The Six Sigma DMAIC process—Define, Measure, Analyze, Improve, Control—is an improvement system for existing processes falling below specification and looking for incremental improvement. The Six Sigma DMADV process—Define, Measure, Analyze, Design, Verify—is an improvement system used to develop new processes or products at Six Sigma quality levels. It can also be employed if a current process requires more than just incremental improvement The Six Sigma LEAN (which is the concept of adding speed to the Six Sigma process) has a tool set that is geared to improve process flow. Six Sigma was designed to specifically focus on process variation (Six Sigma, 2011).

Although there is no single prescription for what currently ails the healthcare system, methods such as Six Sigma can be instrumental in driving change from a grassroots perspective. It can map out targeted areas for improvement and separate larger issues into well-scoped projects that can be effectively measured and managed.

Case Simulation: A high-volume surgical hospital found through a systemwide assessment analyzing opportunities for improvement that perioperative services could be more efficient, with fewer delays and higher satisfaction among the surgeons and operating room (OR) nurses. Revamping the entire department at once would be impractical, costly, and likely to alienate staff and patients.

Instead, the Six Sigma scoping process was used to focus on the critical issues causing the most trouble. Using mapping tools, the Six Sigma Master Black Belt, a person designated as one who demonstrates proficiency in statistical tools and expertise in leading and teaching others, was engaged to understand the flow of work, information, and people. The Black Belt asked the following:

- ▶ *Are the first OR cases of the day consistently starting on time?*
- ▶ *Do the current travel patterns for caregivers and patients make sense?*
- ▶ *Is available space being utilized in the best way?*
- ▶ *Are supplies accessible when and where needed?*
- ▶ *Does the registration or patient preparation process need to be streamlined?*

By diligently gathering data and listening to the voice of the customer, the team was able to answer such questions, zero in on the most critical aspects, and prioritize their improvement efforts. Leveraging Six Sigma techniques, while also working through each phase of the DMAIC process, ultimately led to faster turnaround times, fewer bottlenecks, and less frustration for providers and patients.

ACCREDITATION

Accreditation serves as a symbol of excellence in the healthcare industry and provides an alternative avenue for providers to demonstrate compliance with state and federal requirements. The public and policymakers across the country and in the nation's capital have recognized the value of private accreditation to promote cost efficiency and to ensure that all patients receive high-quality health care. The value of accreditation is widely recognized by all stakeholders in the healthcare arena, including regulators, legislators, consumers, employers, healthcare providers, health insurers, purchasers, and workers' compensation carriers.

Value of Accreditation to Regulators

Accreditation serves regulators in a variety of valuable ways. It

- ▶ Enables regulators to focus limited agency resources on problematic areas identified in audits,
- ▶ Provides regulators with helpful documentation,
- ▶ Facilitates use of current best practices as quality measures because standards are regularly updated,
- ▶ Keeps pace with healthcare advancements more readily than if changes were undertaken by legislation and regulation, and
- ▶ Offers a cost-effective supplement to state oversight of entities' compliance with state regulations.

Value of Accreditation to Legislators

- ▶ Ensures that consumer protection and patient safety are incorporated into operations
- ▶ Drives improvements in health care as a consequence of an impartial and rigorous evaluation process
- ▶ Guarantees that healthcare quality standards reflect the national scope of experience
- ▶ Supports ongoing quality improvement by continually adjusting benchmarks to reflect best practices
- ▶ Provides transparency and accountability through nationally recognized and publicly available standards

Value of Accreditation to Consumers

- ▶ Affords assurance that consumers receive due process (e.g., patient appeals process)
- ▶ Provides evidence that accredited entities are meeting appropriate standards of care
- ▶ Guarantees that confidential information is appropriately and securely handled
- ▶ Sets forth a standard of comparison in evaluating which entities best suit consumer needs
- ▶ Incorporates consumer perspectives into the standards development process

Value of Accreditation to Healthcare Providers

▶ Promotes appropriate clinical oversight of clinical processes

▶ Ensures same-specialty peer-to-peer decision-making for physicians engaged in dispute resolution

▶ Incorporates provider protections and ensures a fair and timely credentialing process

▶ Complements national professional standards of practice

▶ Gives providers a voice throughout the healthcare system

Value of Accreditation to Health Insurers and Medical Management Organizations

▶ Allows multistate entities to meet different states' requirements through a single accreditation process

▶ Differentiates among health insurers, giving accredited companies a marketing advantage

▶ Encourages operational efficiencies that often improve results and reduce costs

▶ Provides evidence that the insurer is keeping current with latest quality benchmarks and best practices

▶ Reduces liability as an effective risk management tool through conformity with national standards

Value of Accreditation to Employers

▶ Provides a measure of comparison in selecting healthcare vendors for employees

▶ Reduces employer-purchasers' burden of oversight of healthcare vendors' operations

▶ Delivers a human resources benefit to employee-consumers who value the "seal of approval"

▶ Promotes the delivery of high-quality health care to employees and provides access to performance data

▶ Helps reduce disability and lost time through conformity with medical management standards (URAC, 2012a)

Today, various accrediting bodies have replaced or work in conjunction with quality improvement organizations (QIO). Organizations such as The Joint Commission, the National Committee for Quality Assurance (NCQA), and the Utilization Review Accreditation Commission (URAC) Accreditation HealthCare Commission are major organizations that provide high-quality peer-review oversight for health plans and healthcare organizations. These accreditation bodies require policies and procedures to be established to ensure that the care provided to patients meets high standards, and that healthcare professionals who provide care maintain competencies that can be measured and reported to the public.

Case management professionals play an important role in assisting their organizations and institutions to meet standards set by these organizations.

CORE MEASURES

As the healthcare industry became more sophisticated in the way it collected, analyzed, evaluated, and applied data, it became more important find a way to measure the same things in the same way. Because the government is a major payer in this arena, it is not surprising that it took this project on. Through the Balanced Budget Act (BBA) of 1997 and the subsequent Balance Budget Refinement Act of 1999 (BBRA), Centers for Medicare and Medicaid Services (CMS) was given the authority to establish and oversee a program that allows private, national accreditation organizations to "deem" whether or not a Medicare Advantage organization is compliant with certain Medicare requirements. Six areas are considered: quality assurance, antidiscrimination, access to services, confidentiality and accuracy of enrollee records, information on advance directives, and provider participation rules. To be approved to make such judgments, an accrediting organization must demonstrate that its program meets or exceeds the Medicare requirements for which it is seeking the authority to deem compliance. Many organizations familiar to nurse case managers met these criteria. Two of these organizations are especially well known: The Joint Commission, formerly The Joint Commission on Accreditation of Healthcare Organizations (JCAHO), and the National Committee for Quality Assurance (NCQA). Both are discussed later in this chapter.

CMS, together with The Joint Commission, worked with hospitals to collect or abstract quality measures. It was expected that hospitals would use these data for their own internal quality assurance as a means to improve the process of care delivered to Medicare beneficiaries. CMS established core measures, and today many organizations refer to these measures as they establish their own, internal core measures for performance in standardization and process management as part of their continuous quality improvement and to meet the clinical measures criteria.

The Joint Commission–CMS Core Measures dashboard includes:

► Substance use
► Tobacco treatment

- ▶ Venous thromboembolism
- ▶ Pneumonia measures
- ▶ Immunization
- ▶ Acute myocardial infarction
- ▶ Children's asthma care
- ▶ Heart failure
- ▶ Surgical care improvement project
- ▶ Hospital-based inpatient psychiatric services
- ▶ Perinatal care
- ▶ Stroke
- ▶ Hospital outpatient department (Joint Commission, 2012)

HEALTHCARE EFFECTIVENESS DATA AND INFORMATION SET

The Healthcare Effectiveness Data and Information Set (HEDIS) is a set of standardized performance measures designed to ensure that the public has the necessary information to reliably compare the performance of managed healthcare plans. The term HEDIS (which originally stood for the Health Employee Data Information Set) originated in the 1980s as a product of a group of forward-thinking employers and quality experts, and was entrusted to the National Committee for Quality Assurance (NCQA); NCQA became the accrediting entity, and is discussed in greater detail later in this chapter. More recently, NCQA expanded the size and scope of HEDIS to include measures for physicians, PPOs, and other organizations, and changed the name to the Healthcare Effectiveness Data and Information Set. HEDIS is one of the most widely used set of healthcare performance measures in the United States. Each year, NCQA makes changes to HEDIS. New measures are introduced, some are revised, and still others are retired.

HEDIS includes an average of 80 measures across five domains of care:

- ▶ Effectiveness of Care (e.g., childhood immunization status)
- ▶ Access/Availability of Care (e.g., adult access to preventive and ambulatory health services)
- ▶ Experience of Care (e.g., member satisfaction survey)
- ▶ Utilization and Relative Resource Use (e.g., frequency of ongoing prenatal care)
- ▶ Health Plan Descriptive Information (e.g., board certification and residency completion rate)

HEDIS represents value on two fronts. First, its measures give the public an unprecedented ability to understand how well health plans are achieving the results that matter. In addition, HEDIS measures ensure results will be comparable across health plans. All measures have three attributes: relevance, scientific soundness, and feasibility (NCQA, 2011a).

Case Simulation: A nurse case manager working for a health plan is interested in the plan scoring well in all HEDIS measures. She is in a position to have an impact on several of the measures, including the rate of eye exams for members with diabetes. To improve this measure, she can reach out to the members in her diabetes disease management program by sending out educational materials on the importance of eye exams. She can further encourage members to seek out this service by assisting them in making appointments and perhaps arranging transportation to an eye care provider. Increased utilization of these services among the members in this diabetes program results in a higher rate of compliance with this standard of care measure and, therefore, a higher score on this measure for the plan.

Patient-centered medical home: The patient-centered medical home (PCMH) is a healthcare setting that facilitates partnerships between individual patients and their personal physicians and, when appropriate, the patient's family. Care is facilitated by registries, information technology, health information exchange, and other means to ensure that patients get the indicated care when and where they need and want it in a culturally and linguistically appropriate manner. Today, many case managers are being embedded in PCMH to help redesign practices to better accommodate the care of patients in an effective, timely, cost-effective, and interoperable manner.

NCQA's Patient-Centered Medical Home (PCMH) 2011 is an innovative program for improving primary care. In a set of standards that describe clear and specific criteria, the program gives practices information about organizing care around patients, working in teams, and coordinating and tracking care over time (NCQA, 2011b).

National Quality Forum (NQF)

The National Quality Forum (NQF) is a not-for-profit membership organization created to develop and implement a national strategy for standardizing healthcare quality measurement and reporting. It was established in 1999 as a public-private partnership through a presidential commission recommendation in 1998, which called for the creation of a national forum in which health care's many stakeholders could together find ways to improve the quality and safety of American health care. NQF does this by

▶ Building consensus on national priorities and goals for performance improvement and working in partnership to achieve them,

▶ Endorsing national consensus standards for measuring and publicly reporting on performance, and

▶ Promoting the attainment of national goals through education and outreach programs (NQF, 2011)

Since then, NQF has not only endorsed performance measures, but also endorsed other types of consensus standards, including preferred practices and measurement frameworks.

It is important for nurse case managers to understand that The Affordable Care Act (ACA) created new responsibilities for NQF as the consensus-based entity. The act charged NQF with convening a multistakeholder group to provide annual input to the Department of Health and Human Services. To accomplish this, the NQF convened the National Priorities Partnership (NPP). The NPP is a collaborative effort of 51 major national organizations that brings together public- and private-sector stakeholders by groups in a forum that balances the interests of consumers, purchasers, health plans, clinicians, providers, communities, states, and suppliers in achieving the aims of better care, affordable care, and healthy people and communities.

NQF has broad participation from all parts of the healthcare system, including national, state, regional, and local groups representing consumers, public and private purchasers, employers, healthcare professionals, provider organizations, health plans, accrediting bodies, labor unions, supporting industries, and organizations involved in healthcare research or quality improvement. Together, the organizational members of NQF work to promote a common approach to measuring healthcare quality and fostering systemwide capacity for quality improvement by setting national priorities and goals for performance improvement, endorsing national consensus standards for measuring and publicly reporting on performance, and promoting the attainment of national goals through education and outreach programs.

Recognizing that nursing care is critical to the quality of patient care and the success of any healthcare delivery system, and realizing that there was an absence of standardized nursing care performance measures, NQF, funded by a grant from the Robert Wood Johnson Foundation, implemented a project to develop core measures for nursing. This project established consensus on a set of evidence-based measures for evaluating the performance of nursing in acute care hospitals. It also addressed the implementation of these measures within healthcare organizations to improve nursing care and patient outcomes, as well as designated a subset of measures that are appropriate for public reporting. While the project emphasized nursing care in acute care hospitals, the framework for general measurement recognized the need for measures to be compatible across different settings of care (NQF, 2011b).

One example is the Nursing Care Performance Measures project, which resulted in 15 NQF-endorsed consensus standards (see Figure 4–2) for nursing-sensitive care. For "nursing-sensitive" care, these consensus standards include measures of processes and outcomes—and structural proxies for these processes and outcomes (e.g., skill mix, nurse staffing hours)—that are affected, provided, or influenced by nursing personnel, but for which nursing is not exclusively responsible.

FIGURE 4-2.
NATIONAL VOLUNTARY CONSENSUS STANDARDS FOR NURSING-SENSITIVE CARE

FRAMEWORK CATEGORY MEASURE

Patient-Centered Outcome Measures

1. Death among surgical inpatients with treatable serious complications (failure to rescue)

2. Pressure ulcer prevalence

3. Falls prevalence

4. Falls with injury

5. Restraint prevalence (vest and limb only)

6. Urinary catheter–associated urinary tract infection for intensive care unit (ICU) patients

7. Central line catheter–associated bloodstream infection rate for ICU and high-risk nursery (HRN) patients

8. Ventilator-associated pneumonia for ICU and HRN patients

Nursing-Centered Intervention Measures

9. Smoking cessation counseling for acute myocardial infarction

10. Smoking cessation counseling for heart failure

11. Smoking cessation counseling for pneumonia

System-Centered Measures

12. Skill mix (Registered Nurse [RN], Licensed Vocational/Practical Nurse [LVN/LPN], unlicensed assistive personnel [UAP], and contract)

13. Nursing care hours per patient day (RN, LPN, and UAP)

14. Practice Environment Scale–Nursing Work Index (composite and five subscales)

15. Voluntary turnover (NQF, 2012)

National Committee for Quality Assurance

The National Committee for Quality Assurance (NCQA) is a private, not-for-profit organization dedicated to improving healthcare quality. Since its founding in 1990, NCQA has been a central organization in driving improvement throughout the healthcare system, helping to elevate the issue of healthcare quality to the top of the national agenda.

The NCQA seal is a widely recognized symbol of quality. Organizations wishing to incorporate the seal into advertising and marketing materials must first pass a rigorous, comprehensive review and must annually report on their performance. For consumers and employers, the seal is a reliable indicator that an organization is well-managed and delivers high-quality care and service.

NCQA has helped to build consensus around important healthcare quality issues by working with large employers, policymakers, doctors, patients, and health plans to decide what's important, how to measure it, and how to promote improvement. That consensus is invaluable; transforming our healthcare system requires the collected will and resources of all these constituencies and more.

NCQA's programs and services reflect a straightforward formula for improvement—measure, analyze, improve, and repeat. NCQA makes this process possible in health care by developing quality standards and performance measures for a broad range of healthcare entities. These measures and standards are the tools that organizations and individuals use to identify opportunities for improvement. The annual reporting of performance against such measures has become a focal point for the media, consumers, and health plans, which use these results to set their improvement agendas for the following year.

NCQA's contribution to the healthcare system is regularly measured in the form of statistics that track the quality of care delivered by the nation's health plans. Each year from 2006 to 2011, these numbers have improved, healthcare protocols have been refined, doctors have learned new ways to practice, and patients have become more engaged in their care. Those improvements in quality care translate into lives saved, illnesses avoided, and costs reduced. For instance, for every additional person who receives beta blockers after a heart attack, the chances of suffering a second, perhaps fatal, heart attack are reduced by up to 40%.

Accredited health plans today face a rigorous set of more than 60 standards and must report on their performances in more than 40 areas in order to earn NCQA's seal of approval. These HEDIS measures were discussed earlier in this chapter. These standards promote the adoption of strategies that will improve care, enhance service, and reduce costs, such as paying providers based on performance, disease management, physician-level measurement, and leveraging the Internet to give consumers more information.

In addition, NCQA produces a product called Quality Compass, which contains commercial, national, regional, and state averages and percentiles of quality scores for health plans. Quality Compass contains information from all HEDIS measures, including utilization data in the Use of Services domain, and some selected Consumer Assessment of Healthcare Providers and Systems (CAHPS®) rates for plans publicly releasing data (NCQA, 2011c).

URAC

The Utilization Review Accreditation Commission (URAC), an independent, nonprofit organization, promotes continuous improvement in the quality and efficiency of healthcare management through its accreditation and certification programs. URAC offers a wide range of quality benchmarking programs and services that keep pace with the rapid changes in the healthcare system, and provides a symbol of excellence for organizations to validate their commitments to quality and accountability. Through its broad-based governance structure and an inclusive standards development process, URAC ensures that all stakeholders are represented in establishing meaningful quality measures for the entire healthcare industry.

In the late 1980s, there was a growing concern over the lack of uniform standards for utilization review (UR) services. UR is the process whereby organizations determine whether health care is medically necessary for a patient or an insured person. As a result, URAC's first mission was to improve the quality and accountability of healthcare organizations using UR programs. In later years, URAC's mission expanded to cover a larger range of service functions found in various healthcare settings, including the accreditation of entities ranging from integrated systems, such as health plans, to smaller organizations offering specialty services. Now, URAC has more than a dozen accreditation and certification programs.

URAC continues to develop new standards for the healthcare system, to revise existing ones to promote national standards, and to ensure that all stakeholders, including consumers and providers, are protected (URAC, 2012b).

The Joint Commission

An independent, not-for-profit organization, whose mission is "To continuously improve health care for the public, in collaboration with other stakeholders, by evaluating health care organizations and inspiring them to excel in providing safe and effective care of the highest quality and value" (The Joint Commission, 2012), the Joint Commission accredits and certifies more than 19,000 healthcare organizations and programs in the United States.

Its process evaluates an organization's compliance with standards and other accreditation or certification requirements. To earn and maintain The Joint Commission's Gold Seal of Approval™, an organization must undergo an on-site survey by a Joint Commission survey team at least every 3 years. (Laboratories must be surveyed every 2 years.)

The Joint Commission provides accreditation services for the following types of organizations:

▶ General, psychiatric, children's, and rehabilitation hospitals

▶ Critical access hospitals

▶ Home care organizations, including medical equipment services and hospice services

▶ Nursing homes and other long-term-care facilities

▶ Behavioral health care organizations and addiction services

▶ Ambulatory care providers, including group practices and office-based surgery practices

▶ Independent or freestanding clinical laboratories

The Joint Commission also awards Disease-Specific Care Certification to organizations that provide disease-specific care and chronic care services, and an advanced level of certification is offered for chronic kidney disease, chronic obstructive pulmonary disease, heart failure, inpatient diabetes, and primary stroke centers. The Joint Commission also has a Health Care Staffing Services Certification program.

The benefits of Joint Commission *accreditation* include:

▶ Helping to organize and strengthen patient safety efforts

▶ Strengthening community confidence in the quality and safety of care, treatment, and services

▶ Providing a competitive edge in the marketplace

▶ Improving risk management and risk reduction

▶ May reduce liability insurance costs

▶ Providing education to improve business operations

▶ Providing professional advice and counsel

▶ Enhancing staff education

The benefits of Joint Commission *certification* include:

▶ Improving the quality of patient care by reducing variation in clinical processes

▶ Providing a framework for program structure and management

▶ Providing an objective assessment of clinical excellence

▶ Creating a loyal, cohesive clinical team

▶ Promoting a culture of excellence across the organization

▶ Facilitating marketing, contracting, and reimbursement

▶ Strengthening community confidence in the quality and safety of care, treatment, and services

Standards and Survey Process

Joint Commission standards address the organization's level of performance in key functional areas, such as patient rights, patient treatment, medication safety, and infection control. The standards focus on setting expectations for an organization's actual performance and for assessing its ability to provide safe, high-quality care. Standards set forth performance expectations for activities that affect the safety and quality of patient care. If an organization does the right things and does them well, there is a strong likelihood that its patients will experience good outcomes. The Joint Commission develops its standards in consultation with healthcare experts, providers, measurement experts, purchasers, and consumers. The Joint Commission on-site survey process is data-driven, patient-centered, and focused on evaluating actual care processes. The objectives of the survey are not only to evaluate the organization, but to provide education and "good practice" guidance that will help staff continually improve the organization's performance. The Joint Commission's on-site surveys are designed to be organization-specific, to be consistent, and to support the organization's efforts to improve performance

Accreditation by the Joint Commission

- ► Strengthens community confidence in the quality and safety of care, treatment, and services
- ► Provides a competitive edge in the marketplace
- ► Improves risk management and risk reduction
- ► Provides education on good practices to improve business operations
- ► Provides professional advice and counsel, enhancing staff education
- ► Enhances staff recruitment and development
- ► Is recognized by select insurers and other third parties
- ► May fulfill regulatory requirements in select states

The Centers for Medicare and Medicaid Services and The Joint Commission worked together to develop core measure sets for many conditions and processes, mentioned earlier in the Core Measures section.

Quality Check® (www.qualitycheck.org) is The Joint Commission's comprehensive guide to Joint Commission–accredited healthcare organizations and programs throughout the United States. This report provides

- ► Detailed information about an organization's performance and how it compares to similar organizations
- ► The organization's accreditation designation and the effective dates of the accreditation award
- ► Programs accredited by The Joint Commission, and programs or services accredited by other accrediting bodies
- ► Compliance with The Joint Commission's National Patient Safety Goals
- ► Special quality awards (The Joint Commission, 2012)

The Magnet Recognition Program

The Magnet Recognition Program® recognizes healthcare organizations for high-quality patient care, nursing excellence, and innovations in professional nursing practice. Consumers rely on Magnet designation as the ultimate credential for high-quality nursing. Developed by the American Nurses Credentialing Center (ANCC), Magnet is the leading source of successful nursing practices and strategies worldwide.

Benefits of Magnet designation include

- ► Attracting and retaining top talent
- ► Improving patient care, safety, and satisfaction
- ► Fostering a collaborative culture
- ► Advancing nursing standards and practice
- ► Growing business and financial success

In the *Leapfrog Hospital Survey*, the nation's oldest survey comparing hospital performance in safety, quality, and efficiency, Magnet designation automatically earns full credit for Safe Practice #9 Nursing Workforce. This section of the survey scores hospitals on their commitment to staffing with highly trained nurses and putting nurses in leadership positions that allow them substantial input on patient safety issues.

Magnet requires organizations to develop, disseminate, and enculturate evidence-based criteria that result in a positive work environment for nurses and, by extension, all employees (ANCC 2011).

Goals and Guiding Principles

The Magnet Recognition Program advances three goals within healthcare organizations:

- ▶ Promote quality in a setting that supports professional practice
- ▶ Identify excellence in the delivery of nursing services to patients or residents
- ▶ Disseminate best practices in nursing services.

The Magnet Recognition Program also provides consumers with benchmarks by which they can measure the quality of the care they can expect to receive in a particular facility. The quality indicators and standards of nursing practice are the ones defined in the American Nurses Association's *Scope and Standards for Nursing Practice* (ANA, 2011). The program is designed to recognize institutions with strong visionary nursing leadership.

International Organization for Standardization (ISO)

ISO is a not-for-profit organization that develops and publishes standards of virtually every possible sort, ranging from standards for information technology to those for fluid dynamics and nuclear energy. Headquartered in Geneva, Switzerland, ISO is composed of 162 members, each one the sole representative for his or her home country. As the largest developer and publisher of standards in the world, ISO fills the vital role of a medium for agreement among individual standards developers, spreading progress made by one country's local developers across the world to further the goal of standardization (International Organization for Standardization, 2012). The ISO series of standards addressed in this chapter is ISO 9000. This series of standards represents an international consensus on good quality management practices. It consists of standards and guidelines relating to quality management systems and related supporting standards.

ISO 9001:2008 is the standard that provides a set of standardized requirements for a quality management system, regardless of what the user organization does, its size, or whether it is in the private or public sector. The other standards in this series cover specific aspects such as fundamentals and vocabulary, performance improvements, documentation, training, and financial and economic aspects.

Peer Review Quality Improvement Organizations (QIO)

The Centers for Medicare and Medicaid Services contracts with one organization in each state, as well as the District of Columbia, Puerto Rico, and the U.S. Virgin Islands, to serve as that state or jurisdiction's quality improvement organization (QIO) contractor. QIOs are private, mostly not-for-profit organizations that are staffed by professionals, mostly doctors and other healthcare professionals, who are trained to review medical care and help beneficiaries with complaints about the quality of care and to implement improvements in the quality of care available throughout the spectrum of care. QIO contracts are 3 years in length, with each 3-year cycle referenced as an ordinal "SOW."

By law, the mission of the QIO program is to improve the effectiveness, efficiency, economy, and quality of services delivered to Medicare beneficiaries. On the basis of this statutory charge, and CMS's program experience, CMS identifies the core functions of the QIO program as:

- ▶ Improving quality of care for beneficiaries;

- ▶ Protecting the integrity of the Medicare Trust Fund by ensuring that Medicare pays only for services and goods that are reasonable and necessary and that are provided in the most appropriate setting; and

- ▶ Protecting beneficiaries by expeditiously addressing individual complaints, such as beneficiary complaints; provider-based notice appeals, violations of the Emergency Medical Treatment and Labor Act (EMTALA), and other related responsibilities as articulated in QIO-related law (CMS, 2011).

Case Simulation: A case manager is collecting and comparing data to the clinical guidelines—either Milliman or InterQual—with which she is working. According to the information collected, a physician has been overutilizing diagnostic tests. The medical director overseeing the case management department discusses these findings with the physician and suggests ways that he can change and improve practice behaviors. Likewise, the acute care case manager discusses a case with the nurse manager on a unit she covers regarding nursing behavior that is having an impact on effective patient care.

The information that the case manager has documented may at some point be needed for a quality study and may be reviewed by the local QIO. This QIO is an independent, not-for-profit corporation committed to assessing and improving the value of healthcare services received by patients through the use of innovative methods and technologies. In some instances, the QIO is contracted by the department of health (DOH) to perform monitoring and auditing functions for the state.

RISK MANAGEMENT

There is a difference between risk management and quality management: QM emphasizes the prevention of client care problems, whereas risk management attempts to analyze problems and minimize losses after an error occurs.

Obviously, if quality management were 100% effective, there would be no need for risk management. In most institutions and organizations, the risk management department has several functions, including to

▶ Define situations that place the system at some financial risk, such as medication errors or patient falls;

▶ Determine the frequency of those situations that occurred;

▶ Intervene in and investigate identified events; and

▶ Identify potential risks or opportunities to improve care.

Each individual nurse case manager is a risk manager. He or she has the responsibility to identify and report unusual occurrences and potential risks to the proper authority. One method of communicating risks is through incident reporting. Incident reports should be a nonpunitive means of communicating an incident that did or could have caused harm to patients, family members, visitors, or employees. These reports should be used to improve the quality of care and decrease risks. Therefore, for a risk management program to be successful, it should have three major components: risk assessment, risk management, and risk communication.

Risk Assessment

Risk assessment is scientifically based. The process evaluates hazards and the likelihood of exposure to those hazards, and then estimates the resulting health impact. It provides a scientific framework for understanding the impact of a wide variety of variables by considering several key questions:

▶ What are the factors that result in risk to the patient or provider's health and the public at large?

▶ What is the likelihood of harm?

▶ How much harm could occur?

▶ How much could harm be reduced by various intervention strategies?

Several forms of risk assessments exist: qualitative, semiquantitative, and quantitative. Qualitative assessments usually identify high-, medium-, or low-level risk. Semiquantitative assessments are used to prioritize risks in relation to one another. Quantitative assessments are often used to identify and evaluate safety control points or estimate the benefits of various intervention strategies.

Each risk assessment has four parts, as widely recognized in the international scientific and regulatory risk assessment communities and by authoritative bodies, such as the National Academy of Sciences. First, risk assessors and risk managers must clarify the health hazard that is the subject of the assessment and any possible policy options that are under consideration. Next, the risk assessors must evaluate the adverse health effects caused by the health hazard. An exposure assessment must then be conducted to estimate the likelihood that the hazard will be present and at what level. Next, a dose-response model is constructed to figure out at what dose or concentration that hazard will cause illness or death.

In the final step of the risk assessment, known as risk characterization, all of the information gathered during the risk assessment process is integrated to show who is at greatest risk, which variables contribute most to the risk, and which intervention strategies would lead to the greatest reduction of risk.

Risk Management

The risk management phase involves using all of the information gathered during the risk assessment to evaluate policy options. Risk managers consider the results of the risk assessment in the context of other policy considerations, such as cost, feasibility, and the social impact of implementing certain policies. This phase identifies, selects, and implements measures that can be applied to reduce the risk identified during the assessment.

Risk Communication

It is important for case managers to understand the importance of risk communication. It is an integral and ongoing part of the risk analysis exercise, and ideally all stakeholder groups should be involved from the start. Risk communication makes stakeholders—risk assessors, managers, scientists, regulators, and so forth—aware of the process at each stage of the risk assessment. This helps to ensure that the process of and information generated by the risk analysis, which includes the logic, outcomes, significance, and limitations of the risk assessment, are clearly understood by all the stakeholders (World Health Organization [WHO], 2012).

Case Simulation: A nurse case manager identifies a situation she feels is unsafe for patients and staff on her floor. The risk issue she has observed is that the used needle disposal containers have been filled beyond capacity several days in a row. She assesses the risk for injury to staff and possibly patients as high. She takes steps to correct the issue by requesting that either larger containers be installed on the floor or the existing ones be emptied more frequently. The risk manager communicates the change to everyone working on the floor and asks their assistance in monitoring the containers to make sure they are only filled to a safe level. These wise and simple steps were easy to implement and probably saved workers on that floor from being stuck by a dirty needle and having to endure all of the follow-up blood tests and precautionary treatments that could result, reduced the risk of a lawsuit for the hospital if a curious patient accidentally got suck by a dirty needle, and saved the hospital money from lost staff time for laboratory testing, sick days, or both.

QUALITY AND DATA MANAGEMENT

> **"**Data is not information, information is not knowledge,
> knowledge is not understanding, understanding is not wisdom.**"**
> —*Clifford Stoll*

Health information technology (health IT) makes it possible for healthcare providers to better manage patient care through secure use and sharing of health information. Health IT includes the use of electronic health records (EHRs) instead of paper medical records to maintain patients' health information. Data and technical standards are critical to the advancement of the national health information technology (HIT) agenda and to achieving many of the agenda's intended health goals and outcomes. Well-defined standards are the foundation for interoperability among systems and for systems that can fulfill the promise of electronically enabled health care. Harmonizing standards allows different information systems, networks, and software applications to "speak the same language" and work together technically to manage and use consistent, accurate, and practical health information for providers and consumers.

With the help of health IT, healthcare providers will have:

- ▶ Accurate and complete information about a patient's health. That way they can give the best possible care, whether during a routine visit or a medical emergency.

- ▶ The ability to better coordinate the care they give. This is especially important if a patient has a serious medical condition.

- ▶ A way to securely share information with patients and their family or caregivers over the Internet, for patients who opt for this convenience. This means patients and their families can more fully take part in decisions about their health care.

- ▶ Information to help doctors diagnose health problems sooner, reduce medical errors, and provide safer care at lower costs.

Widespread use of health IT can also:

- ▶ Make our health care system more efficient and reduce paperwork for patients and doctors

- ▶ Expand access to affordable care

- ▶ Build a healthier future for our nation (U.S. Department of Health and Human Services, 2011)

Nurse case managers are well positioned to move the country's information technology (IT) agenda forward. They possess firsthand knowledge of how data management can affect patients and the providers who care for them. They work in all areas of the healthcare arena and assume a variety of roles—all of which give them unique insight into the good, the bad, and the ugly sides of our healthcare system. They understand what data are needed to manage the care of patients and the importance of being able to access and communicate that data. They sit at many important stakeholder tables, having input into the process of defining standards, and contribute to the design of interoperable IT systems.

The United States continues to have the highest per capita healthcare spending among industrialized countries. Of course, changing demographics such as the aging population, longer life expectancy, a growing number of people living with disabilities, and rampant low health literacy, as well as medical inflation and medical errors, all contribute to increasing costs. HIT is the critical tool that can significantly reduce medical errors, engage consumers and patients in their own health and care, provide information in a coordinated fashion, and reduce costs. This is accomplished through systems and products that electronically create, store, transmit, and present personal health information for multiple purposes, most notably for patient care.

In this nation's fragmented healthcare system, nurse case managers are often referred to as the glue that keeps the system together. They are the advocates, consultants, coordinators, collaborators, educators, facilitators, liaisons, negotiators, researchers, risk managers, brokers, and mentors. All of these roles are enhanced and made easier and more effective when good data management processes and systems are in place, allowing for the collection, analysis, evaluation, reporting, and application of data. This chapter explains these processes and gives some practical examples. Understood throughout this data management discussion is the importance of data security, the need for information standardization, and the mandate to adhere to privacy and confidentiality legislation such as the Health Insurance Portability and Accountability Act (HIPAA), which is discussed in detail in Chapter 5.

INDIVIDUAL AND AGGREGATE DATA

Data need to be complete, accurate, and timely. The word data is the plural of Latin *datum*. It is used to refer to information that has been organized in certain ways. The terms *data*, *information*, and *knowledge* are frequently used interchangeably. The concepts overlap.

Today, most businesses acknowledge that data (not "love" as the song of old spoke of) make the world go round. Therefore, data management is crucial to the success of any business. Health care is no exception. Data management provides the case manager with the processes and structures to create, capture, analyze, and act on information. It is critical to facilitate data sharing and is seen as an effective vehicle for getting the right data to the right person for the right task at the right time. Good data management helps the nurse case manager

▶ Identify patients who would benefit from case management services;

▶ Stratify patients according to their risk levels;

▶ Make better, more informed decisions;

▶ Coordinate high-quality care in a more cost-effective manner;

▶ Contribute to the intellectual capital of an organization;

▶ Gain insight and innovation produced by the free flow of ideas;

▶ Eliminate redundant processes and streamline operations;

▶ Improve customer service and efficiency; and

▶ Be more productive.

Nurse case managers work with two types of data: individual and aggregate.

Individual Data

Personal health information and demographic data are considered individual data. Patients cannot receive appropriate and efficient care unless clinical information about them is available at the point of care. When a patient's health information is not accessible to providers as he or she transitions through the continuum of care, clinical decisions often are made without full knowledge of the patient's history and health status. The absence of needed clinical information can lead to duplication of tests, which not only increases the costs of health care, but also subjects the patient to unneeded clinical interventions that always carry a degree of risk. Similarly, the absence of needed information could lead to incorrect decisions or medical errors that might result in adverse clinical outcomes. Over time, more advanced electronic health records will have integrated clinical decision support with the latest scientific evidence guiding clinical interventions at the point of care. These EHRs will also contain environmental data that should influence many treatment decisions. Increasing the adoption of interoperable electronic health records will improve both the efficiency and efficacy of care.

Case Simulation: A patient is brought into the emergency room complaining of severe abdominal pain. The patient fails to tell the provider that she was admitted to another area hospital with similar symptoms the week before, where a whole battery of tests were ordered and found negative. The patient also fails to tell the treating ER provider that she suffers from depression. The provider, guided by his best judgment, orders the same battery of tests, only to discover the same results.

Imagine for a moment this scenario if all the hospitals in the area were using systems that were interoperable. That same ER provider would enter the patient's demographic information (name, address, date of birth, Social Security number, insurance identification number, etc.) into the IT system and up would pop this patient's medical history and last ER visit information, even though the visit was at another hospital. The provider could pull up the results of all the lab work, x-rays, and imaging tests and review them. He could see what medications the patient was on or was prescribed. Just think of how valuable this information would be to the provider as he conducted his assessment of the patient and diagnosed what was wrong. More than likely, many of the tests and scans would not need to be repeated, the provider could reach a diagnosis faster, and the patient could receive the appropriate treatment. In this instance, the patient benefits, the provider benefits, and the healthcare system in general benefits.

Aggregate Data

Aggregate data, on the other hand, is used to look at populations defined by a common variable or variables, such as disease state or demographic information. *Aggregate data describes data combined from several measurements* or a multitude or combination of other, more individual data. For example, aggregate data can help a nurse case manager identify all patients with diabetes, all patients who are female, or all patients living within a certain zip code. This type of information can usually help a case manager better manage her resources and target her interventions.

Case Simulation: A nurse case manager was asked by administration to join a work group that is looking at patient incentives. This group wants to come up with an incentive program that will encourage adolescents to go to their primary care providers (PCPs) for well visits. In order to do this, the case manager must first understand who the target population is. In this case, it is adolescents between the ages of 12 and 21 who have not received well-child visits in the past 12 months.

Thanks to the company's well-designed database, this information is easily accessible. The case manager asks for a report listing all of the members within the age range who have not had a well-child visit in the past 12 months, and the names and contact information for both the member and the assigned PCP. She then sorts the report by the members' PCPs, and sends copies to the providers, asking them to reach out to these members, or to the guardians for patients under 18, as reminders of the importance of well visits. At the same time, the nurse case manager reaches out to these members directly with a letter offering them an incentive—a free subscription to a popular teen magazine—if they see their PCPs for a well visit before December 31.

This is an example of reaching out to an aggregate population. Of course, the case manager could decide to reach out to an individual adolescent on this list in an effort to encourage the member to see his or her provider, and the case manager could obtain individual personal health information as well.

Whether looking at individual or aggregate data, the steps in data management are the same: collection, analysis, evaluation, reporting, and application. However, the tools used for each process often differ.

DATA COLLECTION

Case managers collect data from a variety of sources—from the patients themselves through a one-to-one encounter either in person or telephonically; from providers and other members of the care team; from the family; or through IT systems such as pharmacy, lab, and radiology databases or enrollment and claims payment systems. These data are then analyzed and the case manager develops a plan of care for the patient. Outcome data is then evaluated and reported, and the information learned is applied to other patients with similar profiles or to make adjustments to the plan of care.

Whether data are collected on an individual or in the aggregate, or collected for personal use or a formal study, it must be collected in an organized fashion in order to be managed effectively. It must be complete, accurate, and timely. It must be "good" data; the data collected must be reliable (results are repeated with subsequent measurements), unbiased (the data contain no systematic errors that either add to or subtract from the true values), and valid (the data measure what they're supposed to measure).

Before data collection begins, everyone should agree on why the data are being collected, what data are to be collected (all the elements and criteria), how they are to be collected, and over what period of time. Once these questions are decided, data collection tools are identified. The case manager may choose a standardized tool or set of tools that have been validated, or develop tools in-house. When doing the latter, it is important to include the end users in the process. Their participation will lead to a more user-friendly and effective tool, with a faster rate of adoption by the end user. It's important that the purpose of the data collection be clearly defined and disseminated before the process begins. Nurse case managers today work in a variety of care settings, including acute, episodic, postacute, subacute, rehabilitation, community- and home-based health care, and the insurance and managed care arenas. These settings and the target population usually determine whether the data the nurse case manager needs to collect is individual or aggregate.

Individual Data Collection

Many case managers today collect data on individual patients using some version of an electronic case management system, electronic medical record (EMR), or electronic health record (EHR) or registry. Some case managers, however, use Microsoft Excel spreadsheets or Access databases, while still others use paper to manage the care of their patients.

President Barack Obama has called for most Americans to have access to electronic health records (EHRs) by the year 2014. Office of the National Coordinator (ONC) measures progress toward this goal by setting ambitious goals for six performance measures. These measures focus on standards for healthcare data to promote interoperability, progress toward interoperable heath information exchange, and the rate of adoption of electronic health records by physicians across the United States. Health information technology is a critical component in improving the quality, safety, cost, and value of health care offered to our nation's 300 million Americans.

E-prescribing and registries have made greater strides in the electronic healthcare arena, with a slightly higher rate of adoption. E-prescribing is an electronic prescribing system that allows the provider to write a prescription on a computerized system and have it electronically transmitted to the pharmacy. Some models of e-prescribing also alert the provider to adverse drug interactions, generic alternatives, whether or not the patient's health plan has the drug on formulary and, in some instances, if the drug requires preauthorization by the insurer.

Registries are systems used to collect and track individual patient information, but also aggregate data pertaining to patient populations with particular chronic diseases.

Aggregate Data Collection

Many nurse case managers working in disease management programs, the public health arena, epidemiology, on research projects, and so forth, use aggregate data. This collection usually involves voluminous amounts of data. Therefore, IT operation systems are used along with software packages and applications to handle the vast amounts of data. These systems are bountiful in the marketplace today and are used by case managers to manage data.

An application, or application program, is a software program that runs on a computer. EMRs, EHRs, case management systems, registries, Web browsers, e-mail programs, word processors, games, and utilities are all examples of applications. The word *application* is used because each program has a specific application for the user. For example, a case management application can help a case manager track her patients and their progress, while a video game can prevent that same case manager from getting the tracking done.

In contrast, system software consists of programs that run in the background, enabling applications to run. These programs include assemblers, compilers, file management tools, and the operating system itself. Applications are said to run on top of the system software, since the system software is made up of "low-level" programs. While system software is automatically installed with the operating system, users can choose which applications they want to install and run on their computers.

Each organization has different needs that require unique software applications. It is important to remember that it is not necessary to understand how each application works; rather, it is important to have a clinical knowledge base to ensure that information reported is logical to the healthcare process. Knowledge is the fuel that allows software applications to work. Commercial applications available include programs such as Excel and Access. These programs allow information to be collected and incorporated into charts or databases to analyze and present information in an organized manner.

Several organizations prefer to customize their own programs rather than buy ready-made systems. Some have IT departments that develop applications to meet the needs of the organization. If this is not available, an alternative is for the organization to contract with consultants who specialize in software development. Understanding and communicating what the needs are and what the organization wishes to accomplish are critically important to the overall success of the process. Accordingly, case managers must take an active role in defining and communicating their unique needs when making application or system decisions.

Data collected using these tools are stored in a data warehouse. A *data warehouse* is a repository of an organization's computer-generated data that is set up in a way to facilitate fast retrieval of correct data without slowing down the operational systems of the organization. Having all data stored in a system that uses standard programming languages and logic to define an organization's business rules is essential if the organization is going to operate from one single point of truth for data.

DATA ANALYSIS

An important step in data management is data analysis. After the data are collected, organized, and summarized, they are put through the process called analysis. *Analysis is the means of looking at data with the intent to extract useful information and develop conclusions.* When discussing aggregate data, the term *data mining* may also be used. Data mining tends to focus on larger data sets, with less emphasis on making inference, and often uses data that were originally collected for a different purpose. Today, the demand for data is tremendous, and in some areas we have more data than we know what to do with. Therefore, data must be analyzed to be useful.

The marketplace is demanding that healthcare providers and payers develop and provide data to improve care, support and define costs, and demonstrate outcomes. To do this, analysis of pertinent data generated every day by all involved in the healthcare system is necessary. IT systems allow organizations to obtain information and generate reports on a variety of topics from the data collected.

If a quality management team wants to evaluate the effectiveness of a particular treatment guideline or critical pathway, data generated from those using the pathway are analyzed to determine variances in care and outcomes that may have occurred. Information gathered from analysis of these areas allows the healthcare team to determine whether the guideline or pathway being used is applied effectively and meeting the desired goals. Data can also demonstrate whether changes in treatment patterns by providers and ancillary professionals have occurred since the guideline or pathway was implemented. Similarly, if an issue is uncovered or an opportunity for change or improvement is identified, a *root cause analysis* is conducted. This is a process used by healthcare providers and administrators to identify the cause or causal factors contributing to variation in performance and outcomes.

The choice of analysis is just as important as any other aspect of data management. A proper analysis should be planned in advance, during the design phase of the case manager's project. Nurse case managers need to ask themselves, "After the data are analyzed, will I be able to answer the question that I set out to answer?"

The basic types of statistical analyses include confidence intervals (used when trying to estimate a population value or the difference between two population values), hypothesis tests (used when testing a claim, such as whether one drug is more effective than another), and correlation and regression analysis (used to show if and/or how one variable can predict or cause changes in another variable).

When analyzing data, it is helpful to display the data. The main purpose of the display is to make a certain point clearly and effectively. The most common types of data displays are pie charts, bar graphs, histograms, tables, and time charts.

Pie charts display data in a circle or pie, and divide the data into slices. They are easy to read and can quickly make a point. A pie chart takes categorical data and breaks them down by group, showing the percentage falling into each group. The sum of all the slices of the pie should equal 100% (see Figure 4–3).

Case Simulation: A hospital administrator is given a yearly report that tells him how many admissions the hospital had in a given year. Realizing that these are important data, the administrator wants to analyze them to see what types of admissions the hospital has so he can determine his budget for the different units and identify any opportunities for improvement. The report tells him that there were 15,350 admissions over the course of the measurement year. It breaks the data down further to read 4,000 admissions for maternity, 8,000 for medical, 800 for psychiatry, and 2,550 for surgery. A clearer, more effective way to display this data is a pie chart.

FIGURE 4-3.
SAMPLE PIE CHART: HOSPITAL ADMISSIONS BROKEN DOWN BY TYPE

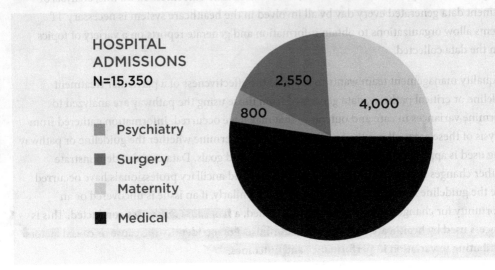

HOSPITAL
ADMISSIONS
N=15,350

2,550

4,000

800

■ Psychiatry

■ Surgery

■ Maternity

■ Medical

Bar graphs are also popular data displays. They, too, use categorical data and break them down by groups to show how many (numerical) or what percent are in a group by the length of the bar (see Figure 4–4).

Case Simulation: An organization working hard to educate both its providers and members about the importance of lead testing for children under 2 years old implemented several outreach strategies, complete with incentives for the providers and the children. In order to determine if the outreach project was effective, the plan collected and recorded data on each 2-year-old as to whether he or she was screened for lead poisoning. A look at 3 years of data showed that in year 1, the plan's Healthcare Effectiveness Data and Information Set (HEDIS) score was 70%; in year 2, the score was 79%; and in year 3, it was 81%. The plan compared these scores to the statewide average (SWA) for this measure, 75%. An easy, clear and effective way to analyze this data is to put it in a bar graph.

FIGURE 4–4.
SAMPLE BAR GRAPH: LEAD SCREENING OF 2-YEAR-OLDS

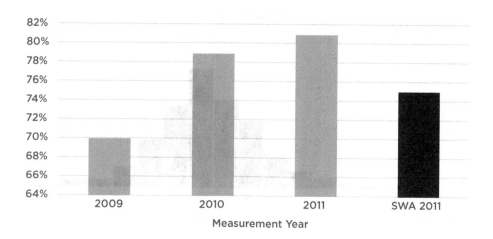

Histograms are bar graphs used to display numerical data (see Figure 4–5). The categories are ordered from smallest to largest. Bars on a histogram touch each other in order to capture each number. Histograms look at frequency (number of patients in each group) and relative frequency (percentage of patients in each group). When histograms are used, they reveal the so-called shape of the data, such as bell-shaped. Do the data look like a mound with tails trailing off to each side? This usually tells the case manager that most of the patients in the sample fall somewhere in the middle of the numbers. For example, if a case manager graphed the average number of days patients stayed in the hospital over a period of a year and the peak of the mound was between 3 and 5 days, with the tail to the left at less than 1 day and a tail at the right at greater than 15 days, then it is visually clear that the two "tails" represented outliers in the patient population.

FIGURE 4-5.
SAMPLE HISTOGRAM: AVERAGE LENGTH OF STAY

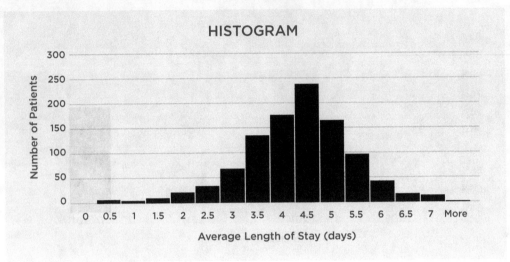

Tables are used to display summary information from a data set. Their column and row formats are clear and easy to read. Unlike a pie chart or graph, a table can show several data points at once (see Table 4-1).

Case Simulation: *If a workers' compensation vendor wanted to understand where it stood financially, it might look to develop a report that told a number of variables: (1) the source of the information (which data system or data warehouse was the information pulled from); (2) the year the claims were billed and paid; (3) the claim type, institutional (inst) or professional (prof); (4) the number of claims of each type for each year; (5) the amount billed for the service; (6) the amount paid; and (7) the totals for each category.*

In this instance, the most effective way to display a report with this many data points is a table. It is clear and easy to understand, and tells the reader immediately what he or she wants to know.

TABLE 4-1.
SAMPLE TABLE: WORKERS' COMPENSATION REPORT

CLAIM SOURCE	YEAR	CLAIM TYPE	NO. OF CLAIMS	BILLED	PAID
Diamond	2010	INST	23,625	$35,025,382	$21,655,827
Diamond	2010	PROF	685,947	$77,890,071	$32,589,359
Diamond	2011	INST	27,671	$49,548,883	$27,620,208
Diamond	2011	PROF	903,422	$115,927,684	$43,292,617
Diamond	2012	INST	28,917	$63,128,150	$30,515,106
Diamond	2012	PROF	1,064,476	$144,500,481	$52,124,815
Grand Total			**2,734,058**	**$456,020,631**	**$197,797,932**

Time charts display data over a period of time and employ a quantity (vertical) axis and a time (horizontal) axis (see Figure 4–6).

Individual data analysis is used by case managers to stratify the acuity level of patients and prioritize case loads. Stratification is used to determine a patient's level of need and is categorized to direct a patient to the appropriate level of case management services, including frequency of contact. An effective case management program should have a stratification process in place that has the following key characteristics:

▶ Methods to map level of needs to case management services and reasonably clear descriptions of the levels to allow all case managers to accurately distinguish levels and apply them consistently

▶ Factors into assignment of case load the complexity of coordination, intensity of services, and frequency of contact

▶ Leads to the intensity of health services coordinated by the case manager in the care plan

▶ Fluidity during the duration of case management (Gesten, Leonard, & Schettein, 2006)

Individual data are also used to assess how a patient is progressing and to determine whether he or she is responding or adhering to a plan of care. For example, if a nurse case manager has been collecting data on a patient over time, she may plot that data in a graph or a chart to see how that patient is responding to treatments and interventions. The patient, too, can see how he or she is doing. Someone once said that a picture is worth a thousand words. When data are plotted on a graph, they are easily interpreted and analyzed—especially if the chart has a reference point on it as well.

Case Simulation: A nurse case manager is working with a patient living with diabetes and the patient's provider to control the patient's A1C levels. The patient is responsive to the case manager and has been watching his diet and taking his medications as prescribed. Although the patient admits to falling off both regimens occasionally, he goes regularly for his blood lab work and receives routine reports from his provider. The problem is that the patient rarely remembers exactly what his last report said. Therefore, he is never quite sure how he is doing. He does remember that his A1C level was 12 in the beginning of the year and that it has fluctuated each subsequent month. That is as much as he can recall. It has become very difficult for the patient to keep track of how he is doing. But once the nurse case manager gave the patient a report that plotted these numbers on a line graph, everyone could easily see that his A1C level was headed in the right direction: down. What made the report even more valuable is that the case manager added a benchmark line at 7 on the chart (A1C level recommended in the American Diabetes Association guidelines) to show the patient not only which direction the A1C level should be going, but also how his levels compared to the national benchmark. It is important to note that benchmarks in this instance should come from a reliable source, a standard or clinical guideline, when comparing data to it. These tools and processes are discussed in detail elsewhere in the chapter.

FIGURE 4-6.
SAMPLE TIME CHART: PATIENT'S A1C LEVELS

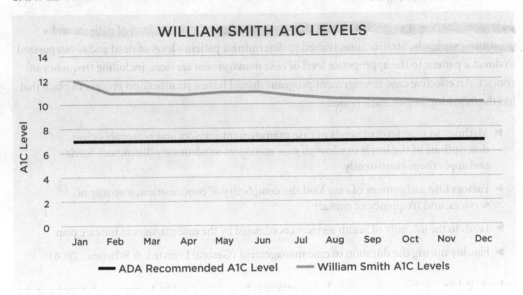

Aggregate Data Analysis

When analyzing aggregate data, statistics are used. A *statistic* is a number that summarizes some characteristic about a set of data. Every data set has a story, and if used properly, statistics do a good job of telling that story. Statistics that are improperly used can tell a different story or only part of it. Whenever data are collected and analyzed, the researcher is typically looking to prove a hypothesis (a claim or its alternative) and determine a significant result. A statistically significant result is one that would have had a very small probability of happening by chance. The *P*-value reflects that probability. *P*-values are used to weigh the strength of the data being used to evaluate the hypothesis. Many organizations do not conduct formal studies but use data analysis to assist in making decisions about how to conduct everyday business.

Case Simulation: A managed care organization (MCO) set out to answer this question: Would hospital readmissions and ED visit rates decrease if members received outreach calls from a case manager after hospital discharge? This was the working hypothesis. However, before the organization made a decision to invest resources and make this outreach service available and ongoing to all of its members, it wanted to see if the hypothesis would prove true. Therefore, it decided to conduct a pilot study. The MCO identified the target population—all members discharged from the hospital during the first quarter of the year (except maternity patients because the MCO already had an intensive case management program in place that routinely made calls to mothers after they were discharged from the hospital). The methodology was also decided: Each member in the target population would receive a call from a case manager. If the case manager was unable to reach the member, a postcard encouraging the member to call the case manager was mailed. A reasonable limit was set for the number of outreach attempts; three phone calls and one postcard attempt would be made before a case was closed with a reason code "all efforts exhausted." A survey instrument was developed for the outreach calls. The survey asked questions such as: Did you receive discharge instructions before you left the hospital? Did you receive any prescriptions for medications and, if so, did you fill the prescriptions? Do you have an appointment to visit your primary care provider, and if not, may I assist you in making that appointment? The case manager's interventions were based on the responses.

The data were collected in a software application program designed in-house by the IT staff. In order to obtain consistent data, the data fields were designed as check-off boxes, yes (y) or no (n), or drop-down boxes. This design would prevent any loss of data, which can sometimes occur when using a free text unreportable field during data entry. In order to analyze the data collected, baseline data were run for the target population and the number of hospitalizations and ED visits for the 6 months prior to the trigger event (hospitalization), and the query was rerun 6 months after the outreach intervention. When the pilot was completed, data were analyzed. The results showed a 12% reduction in hospital visits and an 8% reduction in ED visits. The results were statistically significant and the reduced utilization translated into savings of $450,000 for the MCO. The pilot project was adopted and implemented as a standard service for all members.

Cost–Benefit Analysis

Cost–benefit analysis is used to demonstrate the dollar-spent-to-savings-achieved ratio. In case management, documentation of savings achieved as a result of case management intervention, or as a result of implementation of a service or use of a product, is an important outcome that the case manager can use to demonstrate his or her value to the healthcare system. Components that are included in the cost–benefit analysis are:

► Identifying information regarding the patient

► Overview of the case management intervention

► Summary of the intervention

► Costs associated with the case management intervention

► Any savings achieved. These can include:

  ▸ Avoided charges

  ▸ Discounts or negotiated rates

  ▸ Reduction in equipment and services

  ▸ Gross savings (potential minus actual charges)

  ▸ Net savings (gross savings minus case management fees)

  ▸ Status of case (open or closed)

  ▸ Review of pertinent aspects of the case, including:

    ▹ Clinical

    ▹ Social-situational

    ▹ Educational

    ▹ Wellness

The summary of the cost–benefit analysis should outline the case manager's specific intervention in the case. Issues included are the patient's compliance, enhancement of quality of care, outcomes achieved, prevention of greater illness or injury, and better or more appropriate use of resources.

Case Simulation: An independent case manager is called to work with a 68-year-old woman with peripheral vascular disease who has had four acute care admissions in the past 2 months because of cellulitis The assigned managed care case manager feels that an on-site case manager is needed to find out what factors may be causing the need for frequent admissions. Her supervisor authorizes the contracting of an independent case manager to perform a consultation.

After receiving the referral from the managed care case manager, the independent case manager calls the patient and makes an appointment to see the woman in her home. The patient is found at home, sitting on a recliner with her leg elevated. The case manager notices that the leg is swollen and has an old dressing, which is falling off and is partially covering a large, oozing wound. Several things may be contributing to the poor wound healing and exacerbation of the cellulitis. The case manager observes that the patient lives alone in a small, third-floor apartment and is unable to drive to the store to get the prescribed supplies for her wound care, and, although she has a few supplies from when she left the hospital, she cannot remember how to use them as demonstrated by the hospital nurse. The patient states that she does not want to bother her family since they are all very busy, and admits that she is a heavy smoker, which could be contributing to poor circulation. The patient states she assured her doctor she would stop smoking, but she needs help.

Upon returning to her office, the case manager calls the treating physician to discuss the case. He states that he thinks the patient should be readmitted so that the social worker can find a skilled care facility for her to stay in until her wound heals. Otherwise, he does not know what to do for her anymore. The case manager recommends to the doctor that a course of outpatient physical therapy may be a solution. She states that in her review of the records, the patient's wounds began to heal each time she received whirlpool therapy in the hospital. She suggests arranging for a series of outpatient whirlpool treatments. The case manager also states that the therapy visits will allow professionals to clean and redress the wound, while increasing the woman's circulation as a result of activity. She assures the physician that she will keep him informed of progress and notify him if the wound is not healing effectively so that admission can be arranged.

The doctor agrees to the plan and states he will provide a prescription for whirlpool therapy three times a week, with dressing changes. The case manager uses this opportunity to inform the physician that transportation is a problem, too, and that she anticipates the woman will be compliant with therapy only if she receives dependable third-party transportation, since it is highly unlikely she will contact her family for assistance. The case manager also uses the opportunity to address the patient's smoking. She inquires whether the patient is a candidate for a nicotine patch to help her decrease the number of cigarettes she smokes. The doctor agrees to write a prescription for nicotine patches and third-party transportation for therapy.

The case manager calls the managed care case manager and informs her of the progress, gaining approval to proceed with coordination of the outpatient therapy. Expectedly, the nicotine patch and transportation are denied as uncovered benefits. Anticipating this denial, the independent case manager informs the managed care case manager that she has prepared a brief cost–benefit analysis, demonstrating the expected ongoing costs if the patient does not quit smoking and cannot get to therapy. The independent case manager informs the managed care case manager of the patient's history of refusing to seek assistance from her family, coupled with the other reasons for her repeated hospitalizations. She states that the third-party transportation and the nicotine patches are very small expenditures compared to even one additional hospitalization, which the physician is planning as an alternative treatment.

The managed care case manager delivers the estimated cost–benefit analysis report to her company's medical director, who approves the out-of-benefit items. The independent case manager contacts an outpatient rehabilitation center in the managed care network and close to the woman's apartment that is equipped to provide the prescribed therapy. The case manager inquires about any wellness programs provided by the rehab center and learns that it provides smoking cessation classes. The case manager speaks with the physical therapist, who agrees to plan the therapy to coincide with these smoking cessation classes. The center also provides transportation for its patients.

The case manager speaks to the patient regarding her findings, and the patient is agreeable and thankful for the help. Therapy is scheduled to begin. The case manager follows the patient's progress over the next few weeks. In speaking with the physical therapist, she learns that the patient's wounds are showing signs of healing. The therapist informs her that the patient is attending the smoking cessation classes, in addition to using the patch, and has decreased her smoking from two packs a day to less than a pack a week. The therapist states that she is going to recommend to the doctor in her report that the wound care treatments continue but be decreased to twice a week. The case manager speaks with the patient, who states she is doing much better. She states that this is the first month she is not in the hospital in a long time and is very proud that she is able to cut down on her smoking. In addition, the patient is getting around the house more and should start driving soon.

The treating physician is pleased that the patient is finally making progress. After another month, all treatments are completed, the wound has healed, and the patient is back to her normal activities. The case manager speaks with the managed care case manager and suggests case closure. As part of her final report, the case manager includes a detailed cost–benefit analysis. The report demonstrates that, prior to case management involvement, the patient had four admissions, each lasting about 5 days. The average cost for each admission was $1,800 per day, for a total of $36,000 in a short treatment period, excluding all intermittent physician visits. Care and costs implemented as a result of the case manager's intervention include outpatient physical therapy 3 days a week for 3 weeks, then 2 days a week for 1 month. The cost of therapy was $125 per treatment. The total cost for the outpatient therapy amounted to $2,125. There was no charge for the smoking cessation program or the transportation. The cost of the nicotine patches totaled $145. The independent case manager charged $75 an hour. She included 10 hours of intervention in the cost–benefit analysis, for a total of $750. To recap, the following charges were included in the cost–benefit analysis:

Expenses

► *Cost of physical therapy: $2,125*

► *Cost of nicotine patches: $145*

► *Cost of case management services: $750*

► *Total expenses: $3,020*

Savings Achieved

► *Avoidance of additional 5 days of hospitalization: $9,000*

► *Direct savings for the case: $6,750*

Return on investment (ROI) is one of the latest buzzwords across the healthcare system, with policymakers, payers, and consumers demanding greater value for dollars spent on health care. Government officials, legislators, health plans, and other stakeholders are increasingly being challenged to identify programs with the potential to improve quality of care and control healthcare costs.

ROI is a measure of a company's ability to use its assets to generate additional value for patients and providers. It is calculated as net profit divided by net cost, and expressed as a percentage.

The Center for Health Care Strategies (CHCS) developed a set of tools to help Medicaid stakeholders identify where opportunities may exist to realize both quality improvement and cost containment goals.

One such tool, the ROI/Evidence Base, was developed to help policymakers assess changes in utilization patterns of healthcare costs that may be repeated as a result of specific interventions. Following is an example of a study that proves ROI. Remember that when evaluating studies, it is important to consider the generalizability of published study results to other settings and populations. When using reported outcomes of studies in the ROI/Evidence Base to estimate potential efficiencies of proposed initiatives, case managers should consider similarities and difference in these characteristics: target and sample populations, healthcare delivery environment, intervention implementation, time frames, intensity, financial arrangements, and evaluation design (Center for Health Care Strategies, 2011).

In a 12-month randomized control trial of 937 children between the ages of 5 and 11 diagnosed with asthma receiving care in hospitals and community-based clinics, enrolled to practitioners in private practice in seven inner-city areas in the United States, it was found that by making bimonthly phone calls to advise the children's caregivers on asthma triggers and medication adherence, there was a 24% decrease in the emergency room visit rate and no significant change in unscheduled clinic visits or hospitals (Kattan et al., 2006).

BENCHMARKING

Benchmarking is an ongoing system of measuring products, services, and practices against those of competitors or leaders in a given specialty. It is a process used by healthcare organizations to evaluate various aspects of their processes in relation to best practice, usually within their own industry. This then allows organizations to develop plans on how to adopt such best practices, often with the aim of increasing some aspect of performance. Benchmarking helps a provider improve his or her practice by measuring, evaluating, and comparing both results and processes that produce the best results. It is part of the continuous quality improvement process.

Case Simulation: A facility that specializes in gastric bypass surgery looks at national standards to see how their particular program measures up to other local and national programs. Mortality rates, postoperative infection rates, and length of stay are some important indicators to benchmark in this setting. If the facility ranks high in mortality or postsurgical infection, it will review its internal processes and implement changes that will help lower these rates. After a certain time period, the facility will then reevaluate the data to determine whether or not changes occurred. This process of benchmarking allows the organization to remain competitive in terms of quality, cost-effectiveness, and efficiency.

Best Practice Profiling

The emphasis on quality is a national phenomenon that will only increase in the future. Payers, consumers, insurers, and practitioners are demanding assurance that the care they purchased or received was the best care and as good as the care provided anywhere else by any other provider.

Best practice in the healthcare setting is viewed as a service, function, or process that has been fine-tuned, improved, and implemented to produce superior outcomes. Providers strive to achieve best practices to ensure that the services and products they offer are of high quality and meet consumer, payer, regulatory, and accreditation organization guidelines and expectations. Best practices result from benchmarks that allow organizations to meet or set new standards. They are used to

- ▶ Improve clinical outcomes,
- ▶ Improve administrative efficiencies,
- ▶ Reduce costs, and
- ▶ Provide supportive data in growing market shares and contracting (Case Management Society of America, 2010).

Best practices are not unique to the healthcare industry. Businesses, academic institutions, and other organizations have been incorporating best practices into their structures for a number of years. Throughout the healthcare system, case management is one process being used to promote best practices in healthcare delivery. Effective case management improves the efficacy of care while promoting improved quality of care to gain patient satisfaction. Efforts by case management organizations to define and use best practices within the healthcare environment are an effective way to confront the changes and demands affecting healthcare organizations.

Case Simulation: An area hospital's quality improvement (QI) director noted a significant increase in the number of hospital-acquired decubitus ulcers reported in one of the units. When she brought this to the head nurse's attention, the nurse's reply was, "We have sicker patients on our floor and our nurse-to-patient ratio is higher." The QI director asked the head nurse to stop by her office the following day to discuss the issue further. When the nurse arrived to the QI director's office, charts and graphs were set up around the room. As was said earlier, "One picture is worth a thousand words." In this case, one graph showed the acuity levels of the patients on four units. All were as high as this nurse's unit. Another chart showed the nurse-to-patient ratios for the same four units—again, there was very little difference. Next the QI director showed the head nurse a chart depicting the rate of hospital-acquired decubiti ulcers. When she looked at the chart she could see that her unit was significantly higher than the other three units, and that one of the other units had zero ulcers. After thinking about the data displays for a few minutes, the nurse asked, "So what are they doing on the unit that has no hospital-acquired ulcers?" She wanted that other unit to share their best practices with her. It turns out that all staff on the best practice unit were not only aware of the standards of care in place in the hospital to prevent decubitus ulcers, but one of their staff had actually been on the committee that developed the standards and championed them on her unit. They had regular inservices on the topic, had standing orders from providers for getting patients out of bed as soon as possible, and had special and appropriate diets for persons at risk for developing ulcers. The nurse case manager on the best practice unit offered to share her educational materials and protocols with the nurse from the unit with the high rate of hospital-acquired decubiti. Spurred by the challenge and the embarrassment of not doing as well as her peers, this nurse became the project's champion on her unit and within 6 months achieved similar results.

Best practice and peer review can be very powerful tools.

PREDICTIVE MODELING

Predictive modeling is a data-driven strategy used by healthcare agencies, managed care companies, physicians, and others interested in predicting costs, utilization, and even outcomes when specific variables are applied. This model looks to confirm a correlation between the identification of patients with specific conditions or diagnoses and improved outcomes resulting from targeted outreach efforts. *Predictive modeling* is a process used in predictive analytics to create a statistical model of future behavior. *Predictive analytics* is the area of data mining concerned with forecasting probabilities and trends.

A predictive model is made up of a number of *predictors*, which are variable factors that are likely to influence future behavior or results. In marketing, for example, a customer's gender, age, and purchase history might predict the likelihood of a future sale.

In predictive modeling, data is collected for the relevant predictors, a statistical model is formulated, predictions are made, and the model is validated (or revised) as additional data becomes available. The model may employ a simple linear equation or a complex neural network, mapped out by sophisticated software. (Tech Target, 2012)

Case Simulation: A health plan has used a predictive modeling tool to establish that its patients living with diabetes could be very costly to the plan if the diabetes were not controlled. Therefore, a patient with diabetes is targeted by a nurse case manager for outreach. She contacts the patient to assess his understanding of the diabetic diet, to determine his compliance level, to see if he has equipment to self-monitor his disease, and to find out when his next doctor's appointment is scheduled. The nurse case manager fills in the gaps identified through this assessment to implement an evidence-based diabetes disease management program with this patient. If the patient is willing to participate in this care plan, his diabetes will likely be better managed, his costs will likely decrease, and, more important, his outcomes will likely improve. The intended result of healthcare cost savings should always include improved quality of life and health status for the patient targeted for intervention.

PAY FOR PERFORMANCE

Pay for performance (P4P) programs are now firmly ensconced in the payment system of public and private insurers across the spectrum. More than half of commercial health maintenance organizations are using pay for performance, and recent legislation requires that CMS adopt this approach for Medicare. Simply put, the program is designed to offer providers financial incentives to encourage and assist them in providing the most clinically appropriate care. There are four aspects of P4P program designs that are likely to be of most consequence to individual providers as opposed to group incentives:

▶ Paying the right amount

▶ Selecting high-impact performance measures

▶ Making payment rewards on all high-quality care

▶ Prioritizing quality improvement for underserved populations

Case Simulation: A best practice in the P4P arena is XYZ Health Plan, a prepaid health services plan in New Mexico that serves in the Medicaid and State Children's Health Insurance Program and Family Health Plus Program. XYZ Plan implemented an immunization quality P4P program in which primary care practices are eligible to receive up to $200 per patient. Practices receive incremental dollar amounts for each of the screenings and immunizations administered to children under 2 years old in their practice. As a result, immunization rates for that targeted population increased by 8%.

REFERENCES

American Nurses Association. (2011). *Nursing: Scope and standards of practice.* Silver Spring, MD: Nursesbooks.org.

American Nurses Credentialing Center. (2011). *Magnet Program.* Retrieved from http://www.nursecredentialing.org/Magnet/ProgramOverview.aspx

Case Management Society of America. (2010, June). *Best practice & future trends in hospital case management.* Paper presented at the 20th Annual CMSA Conference and Expo, Orlando, FL. Retrieved from http://cmsa.peachnewmedia.com/store/provider/provider09.php#blank

Center for Health Care Strategies. (2011). *User's guide to the ROI forecasting calculator for health homes and medical homes.* Retrieved from http://www.chcs.org/publications3960/publications_show.htm?doc_id=1261249

Centers for Medicare and Medicaid. (2011). *Quality improvement organizations.* Retrieved from http://www.cms.gov/QualityImprovementOrgs/

Gesten, F., Leonard, M., & Schettine, A. (2006). Seeking to understand case management in New York. *The Case Manager, 17*(4), 55–58, 72.

International Organization for Standardization. (2012). *eStandards store.* Retrieved from http://webstore.ansi.org/SdoInfo.aspx?sdoid=39

Joint Commission, The. (2012). *Core measure set.* Retrieved from http://www.jointcommission.org/core_measure_sets.aspx

Kattan, M., Crain, E. F., Steinbach, S., Visness, C. M., Walter, M. Stout, J. W., et al. (2006). A randomized trial of clinician feedback to improve quality of care for inner-city children with asthma. *Pediatrics, 117*(6), 1095–1103.

Leapfrog Hospital Survey (2012). *Hospital Safety Score.* Retrieved from www.leapfroghospitalsurvey.org/cp

National Committee for Quality Assurance. (2011a). *Summary table of measures, product lines and changes.* Retrieved from http://www.ncqa.org/LinkClick.aspx?fileticket=O-31v4G27sU%3d&tabid=1415

National Committee for Quality Assurance. (2011b). *Patient-centered medical home.* Retrieved from http://www.ncqa.org/tabid/631/default.aspx

National Committee for Quality Assurance. (2011c). *Quality compass.* Retrieved from http://www.ncqa.org/tabid/1402/Default.aspx?q=Quality+Compass

National Quality Forum. (2012). *Nursing-sensitive care: Initial measures.* Retrieved from http://www.qualityforum.org/Projects/n-r/Nursing-Sensitive_Care_Initial_Measures/Nursing_Sensitive_Care__Initial_Measures.aspx

Paton, S. (1993). Fours days with Deming. *Quality Digest, 13 Feb,* 12–16.

Six Sigma. (2011). *New to LEAN Six Sigma.* Retrieved from http://www.isixsigma.com/new-lean-six-sigma/

Tech Target. (2012). *Predictive modeling.* Retrieved from http://searchdatamanagement.techtarget.com/definition/predictive-modeling.

URAC. (2012a). *The value of accreditation.* Retrieved from https://www.urac.org/search/search.aspx?zoom_query=Value+of+accreditation+to+regulators&zoom_per_page=10&zoom_cat%5B%5D=-1&zoom_and=0

URAC. (2012b). *URAC accreditation.* Retrieved from https://www.urac.org/accreditation/

U.S. Department of Health and Human Services. (2011). *CMS and ONC issue regulations proposing a definition of 'meaningful use' and setting standards for electronic health record incentive program.* Retrieved from http://www.hhs.gov/news/press/2009pres/12/20091230a.html

World Health Organization, The. (2012). *Risk communication.* Retrieved from http://www.who.int/foodsafety/micro/riskcommunication/en/index.html

CHAPTER 5

LEGAL AND ETHICAL CONSIDERATIONS

"Good laws make it easier to do right and harder to do wrong."
—William Ewart Gladstone

Nurse case managers are recognized experts in the fields of care coordination, case management, and safe transitions of care. They maintain a patient-centered focus on care while implementing evidence-based interventions to produce the best outcomes for the patient, improve the health of the community, and reduce costs to the system. They are expected to do all of this while remaining an effective patient advocate and operating within the law and their professional scope of practice.

Nurse case managers in their practice are bound by legislation and regulations set forth by the government and held to standards of practice and codes of ethics established by their profession. Therefore, it behooves nurse case managers to be knowledgeable about these laws and the standards and codes set forth by the American Nurses Association (ANA) and the Case Management Society of America (CMSA). In addition, each nurse should know and understand his or her scope of practice.

Before describing some of the laws nurse case managers may encounter and their legal responsibilities, and identifying the ethical issues and principles, let's review what is meant by legislation, regulation, standards of practice, scope of practice, and codes of ethics.

Legislation is law that has been promulgated or enacted by a legislature or other governing body or the process of making it. Another source of law is judge-made law or case law. Legislation can have many purposes: to regulate, to authorize, to proscribe, to provide (funds), to sanction, to grant, to declare, or to restrict. This chapter will discuss more than two dozen laws that nurse case managers should be aware of.

Regulation is administrative legislation that constitutes or constrains rights and allocates responsibilities. In other words, regulations are an interpretation of the law and what you need to do to be in compliance with the law.

Standards of practice (standards of care) are guidelines used to determine what a nurse should or should not do. Standards may be defined as a benchmark of achievement that is based on a desired level of excellence. Standards of care (SOCs) measure the degree of excellence in nursing care and describe a competent level of nursing care.

Scope of Practice. The term scope of practice is used to define the actions, procedures, and so forth that are permitted by law for a specific profession. Practice is restricted to what the law permits on the basis of specific experience and educational qualifications. It is imperative that you know not only your scope of practice, but also the scope of practice of the others who make up a part of your nursing team providing patient care. Remember, if you delegate an activity or task to another caregiver, you remain accountable for the delegation in terms of its appropriateness. Most, if not all, boards of nursing in the United States have information available on their Web sites relating to the laws and rules that govern nursing practice, legal standards, scope of practice, and the like.

Code of ethics. A code of ethics is a succinct statement of ethical obligations and duties of every individual who enters the nursing profession. It makes explicit the primary goals, values, and obligations of the profession. It is the profession's nonnegotiable ethical standard. The Code of Ethics for Nurses is a dynamic document consisting of two components: the provisions and the accompanying interpretive statement.

As professionals, nurses are also self-regulated and accountable for their practice. Therefore, it is important for them to know and understand all applicable local, state, and federal laws. They also need to maintain current knowledge and understanding concerning the scope of practice, patient privacy, and confidentiality; patient rights; requirements for reporting abuse; healthcare proxies; advanced medical directives; patient benefits; and benefit administration, as well as how to utilize appropriate and reliable resources for resolution of legal and other relevant questions—all of which are touched upon in this chapter.

Scope of nursing practice. The scope of practice statement describes the who, what, where, why, when, and how of nursing practice. Each of these questions must be aswered to provide a complete picture of the dynamic and complex practice of nursing and its evolving boundaries and membership. The profession of nursing has one scope of practice that encompasses the full range of nursing practice pertinent to general and specialty practice. The depth and breadth in which individual registered nurses engage in the total scope of nursing practice are dependent on their education, experience, role, and the population served (ANA, 2010a).

The standards of professional nursing practice. These are authoritative statements of the duties that all registered nurses, regardless of the role, population, or specialty, are expected to perform competently (ANA, 2010b).

CMSA Standards of Practice for Case Management

CMSA "Standards of Practice are intended to identify and address important foundational knowledge and skills of the case manager within a spectrum of case management practice settings and specialties" (CMSA, 2010). While the standards are offered to standardize the process of case management, they are also intended to be realistically attainable by individuals who use appropriate and professional judgment regarding the delivery of case management services to targeted patient populations. Additionally, the standards may serve to present a portrait of the scope of case management practice to our colleagues and to the patients who work in partnership with the case management professional.

Two standards applicable to this chapter are legal standards and ethical standards.

ANA standards state, "All nurses are legally accountable for actions taken in the course of nursing practice as well as actions delegated by nurses to others assisting in the delivery of nursing care. Such accountability arises from the legal regulatory mechanisms of licensure and criminal and civil statutes" (American Nurses Association, 2010a).

CMSA's Legal Standard states, "The case manager should adhere to applicable local, state, and federal laws, as well as employer policies, governing all aspects of case management practice, including client privacy and confidentiality rights. It is the responsibility of the case manager to work within the scope of his/her licensure" (CMSA, 2010, p. 19).

An important note in this CMSA standard says

> In the event that employer policies or the policies of other entities are
> in conflict with applicable legal requirements, the case manager should
> understand which laws prevail. In these cases, case managers should seek
> clarification of any questions or concerns from an appropriate and reliable
> expert resource, such as an employer, government agency or legal counsel.
> (CMSA, 2010, p.19)

At this juncture, let me define licensure.

Licensure is an official and legal form of validation required by the profession. Generally, the state government issues licenses and either the state department of education or the state department of health oversees the process. Licenses are issued to ensure that the public will not be harmed by the incompetence of practitioners. Licensure tells the public that the practitioner is knowledgeable and competent and possesses the skills required to practice safely.

While the law may be difficult to understand or interpret at times, resources are available for the nurse case manager to get clarification and education. However, challenges may present themselves in the area of ethics, where sometimes the application of principles in certain situations are not as clear cut, not black and white, and often have many different interpretations.

The following section of this chapter contains brief descriptions of more than two dozen pieces of legislation with which the nurse case manager should be familiar. More in-depth information can be found on the respective Web sites.

Health Insurance Portability and Accountability Act of 1996

Congress enacted the Health Insurance Portability and Accountability Act (HIPAA) in 1996. The purpose of this law is to protect private personal health information from being disclosed to anyone without the consent of the person. Except under unusual circumstances, the consent needs to be in writing.

Exceptions: Some exceptions to the consent provision exist. The consent provision does not apply in the following situations:

- ▶ Treatment
- ▶ Billing
- ▶ Quality assurance
- ▶ Peer review
- ▶ Business planning activities
- ▶ Staff training
- ▶ Required reporting to public health agencies
- ▶ Certain emergency situations
- ▶ Research studies that have obtained a waiver from the Institutional Review Board (IRB)

Research: Private health information can be used in research studies if it is "de-individualized" so that the identity of the individual cannot be ascertained from the information disclosed.

Marketing: Healthcare providers are prohibited from selling or using their patient or enrollee lists to market products from a third party. However, they can use their lists to communicate with or sell their own services to their list members.

Business associates: All business associates, vendors, or other contractors who use the healthcare provider's facility must sign a contract stating that they understand and agree to be bound by HIPAA regulations. A healthcare provider can be held responsible for the actions of the business associate if he or she did not sign a contract, or if there was a history of abuse and the healthcare provider did nothing about it.

Individual rights: Under HIPAA, individuals have the right to

- ▶ Receive notice of the healthcare provider's privacy practices
- ▶ Request restrictions on who is allowed to access their health information
- ▶ Access, inspect, or copy their personal health information

▶ Request an accounting of all disclosures of their health information

▶ Request corrections or amendments to their health information

Healthcare providers' responsibilities: Healthcare providers are required to

▶ Provide security for both paper and electronic personal health information

▶ Institute a complaint process to investigate complaints

▶ Train staff on the law

The HIPAA regulations allow for both civil monetary and criminal penalties for violations of the act (U.S. Department of Health and Human Services, 2011). Components of this comprehensive legislative act include:

▶ Limiting the exclusion period for preexisting conditions mandated by insurance companies to 12 months

▶ Allowing an employee to be automatically eligible for benefits without preexisting conditions when assuming new employment, provided there has not been a break in the employee's group coverage for more than 62 days

▶ Providing for a tax-qualified long-term care benefit

▶ Allowing medical savings accounts (MSAs) on a trial basis for employers with fewer than 50 employees

▶ Providing establishment of the Patient Privacy Regulations, which were released by the Department of Health and Human Services (HHS) on December 20, 2000, and govern the confidentiality of medical records, including electronic records, printouts of such records, paper records, and even oral communications

The Standards for Privacy of Individually Identifiable Health Information (Privacy Rule) establishes a national set of standards for the protection of certain health information. HHS issued the Privacy Rule under HIPAA of 1996. The Privacy Rule is intended to protect the use and disclosure of patients' health information, known as protected health information (PHI) by organizations subject to the Privacy Rule. With the HHS, the Office for Civil Rights (OCR) has responsibility to implement and enforce the Privacy Rule with respect to voluntary compliance activities and civil money penalties.

One of the major objectives of the Privacy Rule is to protect patients' health information while, at the same time, allowing the flow of health information required to provide and promote high-quality health care and to protect the public's health and well-being. Because of the diversity of the healthcare industry, the Privacy Rule is designed to be flexible and comprehensive to cover a variety of circumstances and disclosures that need to be addressed.

Under the Patient Privacy Regulations of HIPAA, healthcare providers and systems are required to implement policies and procedures to uphold the privacy and exchange of PHI data. They are also responsible for training every existing and new employee and member on his or her respective HIPAA privacy policies and procedures. This requirement became effective April 14, 2003, and essentially requires every employee to minimally know the following:

▶ What HIPAA is

▶ Who the entity's HIPAA privacy official is

▶ What the entity's PHI limits are pertaining to patients (what each employee's level of access to PHI information is)

▶ Where to obtain a copy of the entity's privacy notice

▶ What to do when a privacy violation is witnessed

▶ That the care of the patient always takes precedence

Entities and persons required to comply with the Privacy Rule include, but are not limited to, healthcare professionals, pharmacies, hospitals, clinics, home healthcare agencies, durable medical equipment companies, nursing homes, health plans, managed care organizations, employer groups, and even certain government programs that pay for health care, such as Medicare and Medicaid.

Under the provisions of the Privacy Rule, patients have the right to

▶ Obtain a copy of their health records

▶ Have corrections added to their health information

▶ Receive notices explaining how health information will be used and shared

▶ Determine whether to give permission before private health information is used or shared for certain purposes, such as marketing

▶ Obtain a report on when and why health information was shared for certain purposes

▶ File a complaint with a provider, health insurer, or the U.S. government if there is cause to believe that rights are being denied or health information is not being protected (U.S. Department of Health and Human Services, 2011)

Case Simulation: A nurse case manager employed by a managed care organization receives a call from a member who asks for information about the services she has received from a participating provider. The member wants to know what services were approved and when they were approved. The nurse case manager checks the files and tells the member that authorization for a hysterectomy was issued on April 4 of this year. The member thanks the case manager and hangs up.

This scenario sounds harmless enough. However, the case manager violated the Privacy Rule. She did not verify that the person she was speaking with was actually the member. The case manager did not ask certain verification questions outlined in the company's policies to determine whether the person on the phone was indeed who she said she was. These verification questions might include, "What is your name, date of birth, and Social Security number?"

HIPAA created the Medicare+Choice program, which allows new types of health plans to provide healthcare services to Medicare beneficiaries. As of January 1, 1999, any health maintainance organization (HMO) that operated under the prior law and wanted to continue Medicare participation had to contract under the new Medicare+Choice program. Under both the older law and the new Medicare+Choice, Medicare HMOs make annual business decisions about whether or not to participate in the Medicare program. In the Balanced Budget Act (BBA), Congress outlined a payment formula based on a combination of national and local healthcare rates, with an annual minimum percentage increase. Beginning in 2000, payments were determined by blending a percentage of local and national rates and adjusting for the relative health status of Medicare managed care enrollees (CMS, 2011).

Case managers must maintain knowledge of legislation affecting their practices with patients or providers. New legislation and amendments to existing legislation are examples of policy mandates influencing practice.

On December 8, 2003, President George W. Bush signed into law the Medicare Prescription Drug Improvement and Modernization Act of 2003. This landmark legislation provides seniors and persons with disabilities with more choices, better benefits under Medicare, and the first comprehensive prescription drug benefit ever offered under the Medicare program, which is the most significant improvement to senior health care in nearly 40 years. The Mental Health Parity Act of 1996 (MHPA) is a federal law that may prevent a group health plan from placing annual or lifetime dollar limits on mental health benefits that are lower (less favorable) than annual or lifetime dollar limits for medical and surgical benefits offered under the plan. For example, if a health plan has a $1 million lifetime limit on medical and surgical benefits, it cannot put a $100,000 lifetime limit on mental health benefits. The term "mental health benefits" means benefits for mental health services defined by the health plan or coverage.

Although the law requires parity, or equivalence, with regard to dollar limits, MHPA does not require group health plans and their health insurance issuers to include mental health coverage in their benefits package. The law's requirements apply only to group health plans and their health insurance issuers that include mental health benefits in their benefits packages.

If a group health plan has separate dollar limits for mental health benefits, the dollar amounts that the plan has for treatment of substance abuse or chemical dependency are not counted when adding up the limits for mental health benefits and medical and surgical benefits to determine if there is parity.

MHPA applies to most group health plans provided by employers with more than 50 workers. MHPA does not apply to group health plans sponsored by employers with fewer than 50 workers or to health insurance coverage in the individual market. Case managers should check to see if the state law requires mental health parity in other cases.

An example of a coverage provision that violates MHPA is as follows: A plan has a limit of 60 visits per year for mental health benefits, along with a fixed dollar limit of $50 per visit—a total annual dollar limit of $3,000. It places no similar limits on medical and surgical benefits. MHPA does not allow this inequality to exist for group health plans covered by the law.

Group health plans may impose some restrictions on mental health benefits and still comply with the law. MHPA does not prohibit group health plans from

- ▶ Increasing copayments or limiting the number of visits for mental health benefits
- ▶ Imposing limits on the number of covered visits, even if the plan does not impose similar visit limits for medical and surgical benefits
- ▶ Having a different cost-sharing arrangement, such as higher coinsurance payments, for mental health benefits as compared to medical and surgical benefits (U.S. Department of Labor, 2008)

Multistate Licensure

The licensee has the privilege to practice nursing in all states that have adopted and implemented the Nurse Licensure Compact (NLC). The Nurse Licensure Compact allows a registered nurse (RN) and licensed practical/vocational nurse (LPN/VN) to have one multistate license in a primary state of residency (the home state) and to practice in other compact states (remote states), while subject to each state's practice laws and discipline. The NLC allows a nurse to practice both physically and electronically across state lines unless the nurse is under discipline or restriction.

 Advanced practice registered nurses (APRNs) are not included in this compact. APRNs must apply in each state in which they practice, unless they are exempted when employed in a federal facility.

The most current information concerning the Nurse Licensure Compact is found at www.ncsbn. org, using the Nurse Licensure Compact link.

The mutual recognition model of nurse licensure allows a nurse to have one license (in his or her state of residency) and to practice in other states (both physically and electronically), subject to each state's practice law and regulation. Under mutual recognition, a nurse may practice across state lines unless otherwise restricted.

In order to achieve mutual recognition, each state must enact legislation or regulation authorizing the Nurse Licensure Compact. States entering the compact also adopt administrative rules and regulations for implementation of the compact.

Once the compact is enacted, each compact state designates a Nurse Licensure Compact administrator to facilitate the exchange of information between the states relating to compact nurse licensure and regulation. On January 10, 2000, the Nurse Licensure Compact Administrators (NLCA) were organized to protect the public's health and safety by promoting compliance with the laws governing the practice of nursing in each party state through the mutual recognition of party state licenses.

Emergency Medical Treatment and Active Labor Act (EMTALA)

Passed in 1986, this act applies to all hospitals receiving Medicare funds and maintaining an emergency room. Also known as the "patient dumping law," this act requires emergency rooms to screen a patient to determine whether the patient suffers from an emergency medical condition or if a pregnant patient is in active labor before asking the patient about ability to pay or method of payment. If the patient is found to be suffering from an emergency medical condition or is in active labor, the hospital must provide necessary and appropriate treatment to stabilize the patient. The hospital cannot delay treatment to determine payer benefits. In amendments to the law passed in 1989, specialty hospitals (e.g., burn units, trauma centers) must accept transfer of a patient requiring special treatment available at the facility, regardless of the patient's ability to pay. The act also prevents hospitals from admitting the patient and then immediately discharging the patient in an effort to circumvent the law.

EMTALA also governs a managed care company's request to have a patient transferred from a nonparticipating hospital in the managed care network to a participating hospital in the managed care network. Before the request can be fulfilled, the acute care–based case manager needs to ensure that the patient is medically stable for transfer, that the treating physician authorizes transfer, that there is a treating physician willing to accept the patient at the new facility, that the patient has consented to the transfer, and that the patient's medical records accompany the patient at the time of transfer.

While the issue of delegation of care is not a law, it is an important component of EMTALA for the case manager to understand. EMTALA mandates that when a patient is eligible for transfer to another facility for necessary care, legal guidelines determine delegation of care from one facility to another. Internally, healthcare facilities and systems must determine how delegation of care will occur in an ethical and legal manner, and then set policies and procedures to govern appropriate delegation of care. Entire patient management processes are developed and job descriptions molded to ensure that the delegation of care is purposeful and appropriate.

Delegation is a contractual agreement in which authority and responsibility for a task is transferred by the person accountable for the task to another individual. When performed appropriately, delegation benefits the delegator, the delegatee, the organization, and the patient. Appropriate delegation involves all of the following components:

▶ Identifying and determining the task and the who is responsible

▶ Identifying who has the skills and abilities to describe expectations clearly

▶ Reaching a mutual agreement on the assigned task or duties

▶ Equipping the delegatee with the resources to carry out the assigned task or duties

▶ Monitoring the performance of the delegatee and providing feedback when necessary

Adhering to the steps of delegation minimizes the risk of liability for a healthcare professional, particularly if the healthcare professional prudently selects a qualified person as the delegatee and provides appropriate supervision of performance. This is notably true in case management, where delegation of care can also pertain to appropriate assignment of services and products to benefit a patient.

Case Simulation: Case managers sometimes aren't as organized about delegating care once responsibility for the patient reaches their department. Case managers often fail to delegate care once they have initiated a care plan and are coordinating services. Instead of consulting with a dietitian and a social worker for the noncompliant adolescent with diabetes, for example, a case manager might instead try on his or her own to sort through the teenager's anger over being "sick" and refusal to eat the right foods.

Why does the case manager fail to follow through with delegation? Good case management requires the professional to be very proficient. Many case managers have a "just do it" attitude. They try to be all things to all people. Others see delegation as a loss of control. Still others are mistrustful that the task will be completed in a timely and efficient manner by someone else. It is important for the case manager to differentiate those tasks that should be completed by a case manager from those that should be completed by other professionals, the caregiver, or even the patient. The best interests of the patient should be the deciding factor when considering delegation (Powell, 1996).

The Omnibus Budget Reconciliation Act (OBRA) is a broad-based legislative act with many implications. In the 1989 and 1990 amendments of OBRA, individual states of the OBRA Act, individual states are required to provide Medicaid coverage for all pregnant women and their children up to 6 years of age if the family income is less than 133% of the federal poverty level. Also formed from this act was the Agency for Health Care Policy and Research (now known as the Agency for Healthcare Research and Quality), which continues to be an active overseer of managed care and healthcare delivery.

Written in 1990 and enacted in 1991, the Patient Self-Determination Act requires that healthcare facilities in the United States advise patients upon admission of their rights to accept or refuse treatment should they become gravely ill. The following facilities must comply with the law: hospitals, hospice, subacute facilities, skilled nursing facilities, and home healthcare agencies that accept Medicaid or Medicare patients. Under the act, patients are entitled to advance directives— living wills and durable power of attorney proxies. Living wills designate whether an individual desires life-prolonging treatment in the event that he or she is unable to make medical decisions. A durable power of attorney designates who will make healthcare decisions in the event that an individual is unable to make medical decisions.

The act requires healthcare providers to perform the following:

▶ Provide adult patients with written notification of their state law regarding advance directives and the right to refuse treatment, and provide the policies of the facility or agency

▶ Document in the patient's medical record whether he or she has advance directives

▶ Ensure compliance with applicable state laws on advance directives

▶ Create and maintain policies and procedures on advance directives, and educate the staff regarding these policies and procedures

All hospitals receiving Medicare or Medicaid funding are required to establish written guidelines for identifying potential organ donors under the Uniform Anatomical Gifts Act. A potential donor is defined as a person who dies in circumstances that are generally acceptable for donation of at least one solid organ if the donor can be identified in a timely manner, and if permission for the donation is obtained.

Rehabilitation Legislation

Section 501: This section of the act promulgates basic federal law containing programs and civil rights for all persons with disabilities.

Section 502: This section is an amendment to the Rehabilitation Act. It pertains to the governance and accessibility laws provided by the Architectural and Transportation Barriers Compliance Board (ATBCB).

Section 503: This is an amendment to the Rehabilitation Act pertaining to affirmative action for persons with disabilities. Compliance is required by federal employers and entities operating in federal locations or funded with federal dollars.

Section 504: This amendment to the act pertains to nondiscrimination of persons with disabilities by the federal government, entities operating in federal locations, or those funded with federal dollars.

This act established vocational rehabilitation as a permanent federal program in 1935. When people apply under any one of the disability provisions of the Social Security law, they are automatically referred to individual state vocational rehabilitation programs. Agencies and eligibility for services vary state to state. However, states are responsible for providing counseling, training, or other services to support the return of disabled persons to work on a part-time or full-time basis.

This legislation provides matching federal funds to states for vocational education programs that were implemented prior to enactment of permanent programs through the Social Security Act.

Also known as the Civilian Vocational Rehabilitation Act, this legislation provides for the initiation of civilian vocational rehabilitation programs.

Disability Legislation

This has been the most comprehensive, complex legislation passed to date to protect the rights of disabled persons. Broad legislation is defined through five distinct sections, known as titles.

Title I: Pertains to employment provisions and has been enforced by the Equal Employment Opportunity Commission (EEOC) in Washington, D.C., since July 26, 1992. Effective July 26, 1994, companies with 15 or more employees must comply with the mandates of Title 1. (See the Employer Legislation section of this chapter for further information.)

Title II: Pertains to public transportation, providing access to public transportation for all disabled individuals. Enforcement is by the U.S. Department of Transportation (DOT). Examples of mandated provisions include wheelchair lifts included on public transportation (city buses) and on private transportation accessed by the public (car rental shuttle buses).

Title III: Pertains to public access provisions, providing for accessible public accommodations in all settings visited or used by disabled citizens. Title III has been federally enforced since January 1, 1993, by the U.S. Department of Justice (DOJ).

Title IV: Pertains to accessible transmitting and telecommunication devices (TTDs). This affects telecommunications companies and all industries using these devices (e.g., hotel telephones, hospital television sets).

Title V: Pertains to arbitration and allows a legal process by which a disabled person can seek restitution for damages caused by inaccessibility of services.

This act requires federal and federally assisted buildings and facilities to be accessible to and usable by persons with disabilities.

This legislation provides the right for all disabled children to receive "free appropriate public education" and extensive "due process" procedures. The act promotes equal educational opportunities regardless of the child's degree of disability or services needed to achieve equality. It establishes procedures by which disabled children are evaluated and their classifications determined. It then provides for the development and implementation of appropriate programs of special education and "related services" stemming from the evaluations and classifications. These are known as individualized education programs (IEP) and must be developed jointly by school officials and parents.

Social Security Disability Insurance (SSDI) legislation provides for disability insurance, as part of the federal Social Security program, to replace part of earnings lost because of any physical or mental impairment severe enough to prevent an individual from working. Monthly case benefits are paid to eligible disabled persons and to eligible auxiliary beneficiaries (e.g., eligible person's minor children) throughout a period of disability after an initial 5-month waiting period.

The Social Security Act established vocational rehabilitation as a permanent federal program in 1935.

The act provides special provisions for handicapped and elderly people regarding public transportation, and it stood alone as the transportation-related access law until the Americans with Disabilities Act (ADA) was enacted.

Employer Legislation

According to Title I of the ADA, employers may not discriminate against qualified individuals seeking a job offer or holding a job. Employers must reasonably accommodate the disabilities of qualified applicants or employees, including modifying work stations and equipment, unless an undue hardship to the company would result. Undue hardship is determined on a case-by-case basis by the EEOC, through the arbitration process under Title V of the act, or both. Individuals may file complaints with the EEOC or via a private lawsuit after exhausting administrative remedies. Remedies are the same as those available under Title VII of the Civil Rights Act of 1964. The court may order the employer to hire or promote qualified individuals, reasonably accommodate their disabilities, pay back wages and attorneys' fees, or a combination of these.

Additional information about Title I of the ADA that case managers should be familiar with follows:

If a person is otherwise qualified to perform a job, but cannot perform one or more essential job functions because of disability, reasonable accommodation must be made for the disabled employee. Essential job functions are defined by the employer. It is the responsibility of the employer to have written job descriptions and to state all of the essential job functions in each written job description.

A reasonable accommodation is defined as any change in the work environment or in the way things are usually done that results in equal employment opportunity for a person with a disability. Employers are obligated to make reasonable accommodation unless they can show that the accommodation would cause an undue hardship on the operation of the business. Undue hardship is defined as excessively costly, extensive, substantial, or disruptive, or a solution that would fundamentally alter the nature or operation of the business (Americans with Disabilities Act of 1990 as amended).

An example of reasonable accommodation: A disabled employee must have equal access to lunchrooms; employee lounges; restrooms; meeting rooms; and any employer-sponsored services, such as health programs, transportation, and social events.

The Consolidated Omnibus Budget Reconciliation Act (COBRA), passed in 1986, requires employers and their health insurance group plans to provide the temporary extension of health benefits coverage to an employee, the spouse, and any dependent children after the employee leaves a job. Coverage must be offered for a fixed period of time at a predetermined group rate. The employee must be covered under the employer's group health insurance plan in order to qualify, even if the employee is only covered for 1 day at the time of departure from the job. Employers are also required to offer COBRA benefits to divorced or widowed spouses and former dependent children of employees under the act.

The following scenarios qualify as "leaving the job":

- ► Voluntary resignation
- ► Strike or walkout
- ► Layoff or reduction in hours
- ► Termination (not through gross misconduct)
- ► Death
- ► Retirement
- ► Entitlement of the employee to Medicare coverage
- ► Dependent child's loss of dependence by reaching a certain age

COBRA benefits are available to employees and family members for 18 months. However, if spouses and dependents of an employee have coverage as a result of the employee's death, divorce, legal separation, age limitation, or the employee's eligibility for Medicare, spouses and dependents are entitled to 36 months of coverage.

The Employee Retirement Income Security Act (ERISA) of 1974 sets minimum standards for pension plans in private industry. This act applies two types of private employee benefit plans: pension plans and employee welfare benefit plans, which provide benefits in the event of sickness, hospitalization, surgery, accident, death, disability, or unemployment. Of note is that ERISA exempts nongovernmental, self-insured employee benefit plans from meeting the minimum benefit regulations required of other nongovernmental insurance companies. This act serves as the cornerstone of federal worker protection. It provides a minimum hourly wage, requires payment of additional compensation for overtime, regulates child labor, and prohibits working from home in certain industries.

The Fair Labor Standards Act is enforced by the U.S. Department of Labor's Wage and Hour Division. The Family Medical Leave Act (FMLA) requires covered employers to provide up to 12 weeks of unpaid, job-protected leave in a 12-month period to eligible employees for certain family and medical reasons. Employees are eligible if they have worked for a covered employer for at least 1 year and for 1,250 hours over the previous 12 months. The employer is eligible if there are at least 50 employees employed within 75 miles. During the leave, the employer must maintain health benefits for the employee if the employee desires.

However, the employer is not required to pay health benefits beyond the 12 weeks if the employee cannot return to work. In this scenario, COBRA benefits, covered earlier in this chapter, would be assigned. Employees are entitled to work fewer hours per week or per work day if a serious health condition warrants reduction in work time. The employer is entitled to require that the serious health condition be certified by a healthcare provider.

Unpaid leave must be granted for any of the following reasons:

- ▶ To care for the employee's child after birth or placement of a child with the employee for adoption or foster care
- ▶ To care for the employee's spouse, son or daughter, or parent who has a serious health problem
- ▶ To attend to a serious health condition that makes the employee unable to perform his or her job

At the employer or employee discretion, certain kinds of paid leave may be substituted for unpaid leave. These may include short- or long-term disability benefits. The FMLA is enforced by the U.S. Department of Labor, which is authorized to investigate and resolve complaints of violations by the employee or employer.

First enacted in 1928, with amendments in 1972, the Longshore and Harbor Workers' Compensation Act, this act is administered by the Department of Labor through the Office of Workers' Compensation. It provides medical and financial benefits to longshoremen and harbor workers while they are unable to work for various reasons, including job modifications and retraining when the worker is able to resume work. The claims examiner acts as a case manager responsible for the financial and medical direction of the case, and refers the client to a rehabilitation specialist. Vocational rehabilitation is not mandatory under the act.

The Occupational Safety and Health Act establishes the Occupational Safety and Health Administration (OSHA) as the primary regulatory system for workplace health and safety. OSHA rules include numerous safety standards and requirements for employers. They also require employers to maintain injury records and provide employees with information about hazards in the workplace. States are free to establish their own OSHA agencies, provided the safety requirements are at least as stringent as those at the federal level.

In another move to make Medicare the secondary payer behind employer group health benefit plans (see TEFRA below), this act mandates that employer plans are first payer for employees or their dependents who are permanently disabled and Medicare-eligible. As stated earlier in this chapter, OBRA is a broad-based legislative act with many implications. This chapter offers brief encapsulations of specific components of legislation.

OBRA amended the Social Security Act, making Medicare the secondary payer behind employer group health benefit plans for employees and their spouses between the ages of 65 and 69. Under the act, employers were required to offer employees in this age range the same health benefits as those offered to younger employees. However, in 1986, the employer's plan became the primary payer for all active, Medicare-eligible employees and their spouses, regardless of age.

OBRA established a no-fault system that originally provided workers' compensation laws in 10 states. It requires the employer to assume the cost of occupational disability, death, or disease, without regard to fault. All state workers' compensation systems provide wage replacement for both temporary and permanent disabilities, regardless of whether the employer or the worker is at fault for the injury or illness.

Patient Protection and Affordable Care Act

In 2010, the Patient Protection and Affordable Care Act was signed into law. The following summary of the law and changes made to the law by subsequent legislation focuses on provisions of special interest to nurse case managers. The overarching goal of the law is to expand health insurance coverage, control healthcare costs, and improve the healthcare delivery system.

What is in the bill that interests nurse case managers?

▶ Proposed models and financing mechanisms for coordinated care through demonstration and pilot projects

▶ Creation of an Innovation Center within the Centers for Medicare and Medicaid Services (CMS)

▶ Proposal to use a diverse network to improve care coordination for persons with two or more chronic conditions and a history of prior-year hospitalization through interventions developed under the Medicare Coordinated Care Demonstration Project

▶ Establishment of a Community-Based Care Transitions Program

▶ Establishment of community-based interdisciplinary teams to support primary care practices

Title III: Section 3025 — Hospital readmissions reduction program

▶ This provision would adjust payments for hospitals paid under the inpatient prospective payment system based on the dollar value of each hospital's percentage of potentially preventable Medicare readmissions for the three conditions with risk-adjusted readmission measures that are currently endorsed by the National Quality Forum.

▶ Provides the Secretary of Health and Human Services authority to expand the policy to additional conditions in future years and directs the Secretary to calculate and make publicly available information on all patient hospital readmission rates for certain conditions. These conditions include those that are high volume or high expenditure and excludes readmissions unrelated to prior discharge, such as a planned readmission.

Title III: Section 3036 — Community-Based Care Transitions Program

▶ Provides funding to hospitals and community-based entities that furnish evidence-based care transition services to Medicare beneficiaries at high risk for readmission

Care Coordination and Case Management

Title III: Section 3502 — Improving the Quality and Efficiency of Health Care

▶ Creates processes for the development of quality measures involving input from multiple stakeholders and for selecting quality measures to be used in reporting to and payment under federal health programs

Establishing community health teams to support the patient-centered medical home

▶ Creates a program to establish and fund the development of community health teams to support the development of medical homes by increasing access to comprehensive, community-based coordinated care

Program to facilitate shared decision-making

▶ Calls for the establishment of independent standards for patient decision aids as well as a program to develop and update those standards. It creates a grant program to establish Shared Decision-Making Resource Centers.

Healthcare Reform Industry Impacts

Title III: Improving the Quality and Efficiency of Health Care

This section provides incentives for doctors and hospitals that improve quality while providing for better coordination that helps to reduce harmful medical errors and healthcare-acquired infections.

Title IV: Prevention of Chronic Disease and Improving Public Health

▶ This section improves data collection and analysis, facilitates better data sharing, and requires the development of standards for the collection of data regarding the nation's health and the performance of the nation's health care, including health disparities.

▶ Focus on the core areas of interest for patient-centered organizations: care coordination, case management, disease management, and transition of care

National Pilot Program on Payment Bundling

Title III: Section 3023

▶ This section will direct the Secretary to develop a 5-year national, voluntary pilot program encouraging hospitals, doctors, and postacute-care providers to improve patient care and achieve savings for the Medicare program through bundled payment models. The Secretary is also required to submit a plan to Congress to expand the pilot program if doing so will improve patient care and reduce spending.

Demo Project to Evaluate Integrated Care Around Hospitalization

Title II: Section 2704

▶ Establishes a demonstration project, in up to eight states, to study the use of bundled payments for hospital and physician services under Medicaid

State Option — Provide Health Homes to Medicaid Enrollees With Chronic Conditions

Title II: Section 2703

▶ Provides states the option of enrolling Medicaid beneficiaries with chronic conditions into a health home. Health homes would be composed of a team of health professionals and would provide a comprehensive set of medical services, including care coordination.

Establishment of CMS Innovation Center

Title III: Section 3021

▶ Establishes within the Centers for Medicare and Medicaid Services (CMS) a Center for Medicare and Medicaid Innovation. The purpose of the center will be to research, develop, test, and expand innovative payment and delivery arrangements to improve the quality and reduce the cost of care provided to patients in each program. Dedicated funding is provided to allow for testing of models that require benefits not currently covered by Medicare. Successful models can be expanded nationally.

Patient-Centered Outcomes Research Institute

Title VI: Section 6301

▶ Creates a freestanding nonprofit corporation called the Patient-Centered Outcomes Research Institute to assist patients, clinicians, and others to make informed decisions and to identify research priorities and develop an agenda. The Research Project Agenda identifies priorities such as disease incidence, prevalence, and burden in the United States; practice variations; and health disparities. In identifying research priorities, the Institute will take into account disease incidence, prevalence, and the burden of chronic conditions.

LEGAL RESPONSIBILITIES

There are many legal responsibilities that are a common part of case management practice. It is incumbent on the nurse to understand the different laws that affect the practice—and several criminal and civil laws that exist. Two types of criminal laws establish felonies and misdemeanors. A felony is an act punishable by death or imprisonment for greater than 1 year (e.g., murder, failure to report child abuse, fraud in business records, patient abuse and neglect, stealing, selling or using illegal drugs). A misdemeanor is any other type of crime.

Case Simulation: While conducting a narcotics check at the end of her shift, a nurse case manager notices the count is short one controlled analgesic. She finds a patient whose PRN orders allow him to have that medication for pain, but she notices that he hasn't had any in a long time. She signs the missing dose out to that patient, who in reality did not receive that dose. This is a violation of narcotics laws.

Abandonment

Unfortunately, abandonment of patients occurs in many settings and for a myriad of reasons. Abandonment is the willful neglect of responsibility for another person by a person who is assigned to care for that patient or by a person who is in a caregiving position.

Case Simulation: A case manager is coordinating services for a newborn who was abandoned by his parent(s) and requires immediate medical care in addition to urgent application for social services, such as parental foster care and ongoing medical coverage. The case manager or resource manager initially concentrates on mobilizing services to provide the infant with the most basic needs—food, shelter, and safety—while at the same time following the organization's legal procedures pertaining to abandonment, which is in compliance with individual state laws on abandonment. These may include cooperating with local authorities in an attempt to identify one or both parents in order to collect medical or other background information that could be vital to the infant's future well-being.

Similarly, many challenges surround abandoned adults, particularly developmentally disabled adults and older individuals. Adults can be abandoned in their own homes or in adult care homes and facilities, because abandonment does not necessarily mean that a caregiver has permanently left the premises. When an infant is abandoned at a police station by the parent, the intent of abandonment is clear. Abandonment of an older, ill, or injured person being cared for by a third party is more difficult to define. Abandonment should be suspected if

- ▶ The caregiver leaves for a period of time without arranging for substitute care;
- ▶ An employed aide does not show up for work; or
- ▶ A person's care deteriorates markedly, even with the presence of the caregiver in the home or facility (Mitchell, 2007).

At times, case managers may observe older patients or developmentally disabled patients who are transferred to a hospital from a caregiver setting and appear neglected or abused. The patient may have serious bedsores, wounds, bruises, emaciation, or other signs of physical neglect or abuse. Acute care facilities have policies and procedures in place to report any suspicion of abuse or neglect. The case manager should be familiar with these policies and procedures to uphold the rights of the patient, as well as the legal responsibility of the case manager and the facility.

Whether abandonment is intentional or unintentional and what punishment, if any, will be applied, depends on individual state law. Again, it is the responsibility of the case manager to know and understand the law(s) of the state in which he or she practices because each state's legislation is unique. A number of states have passed laws permitting parents to drop off babies at specified "safe places," such as hospitals and police stations, with no questions asked and no penalties enforced. These laws are intended to protect babies who might otherwise be harmed or abandoned as unwanted. Laws pertaining to abandonment of older persons also vary from state to state, and are usually captured under the umbrella of elder abuse.

Reporting of Abuse

Elder abuse and child abuse are unfortunate and often occur in devastating circumstances to which the case manager will likely be exposed from time to time. In addition to the many services the case manager may mobilize on behalf of an abused patient, case managers and all healthcare professionals are legally responsible for reporting any suspicion of abuse. Again, each state varies in the laws pertaining to and the reporting of abuse. Case managers must be familiar with the state laws governing the reporting of abuse for their practices or the state in which the patient resides. They must also be familiar with policies and procedures of their employers regarding the reporting of abuse within a healthcare facility. Reporting of both child and elder abuse is mandatory in many states for *any person* who suspects or has reason to suspect abuse. However, every state and the District of Columbia have statutes identifying mandatory reporters of child maltreatment and under what circumstances they are to report. Persons typically identified as mandatory reporters include all healthcare practitioners, law enforcement or social service agency employees, any dependent care custodian or provider, coroners, and school personnel. Failure to report abuse is punishable.

How and where to report suspected abuse varies according to state law. If a case manager suspects abuse, he or she should have access to the 800-number hotlines to report abuse within all 50 states. This information is readily available in healthcare facilities, such as in emergency rooms of acute care hospitals. Hotline numbers are also available on various Web sites. Elder abuse hotlines for all 50 states are listed online at http://alzheimers.about.com. Child abuse hotlines are listed by the National Clearinghouse on Child Abuse and Neglect Information at http://nccanch.acf.hhs.gov/.

Generally, the same laws that require persons to report abuse also protect individuals from criminal liability for reporting the suspected abuse, unless the person reporting the abuse knowingly makes false statements. The identity of the person reporting the abuse is kept confidential.

Informed Consent

Informed consent has meant different things over the course of time. Throughout history, what the physician said would happen, did, whether the patient agreed or disagreed. There was no questioning the physician's judgment or authority. Only recently has the fundamental right of self-determination been recognized that requires the collaboration of the physician and patient. Legally, it is a well-established principle that all healthcare professionals are responsible for making adequate disclosures of information to a patient and to obtain an informed consent for treatment from the patient. The person who is legally responsible for obtaining informed consent is the person who will provide the treatment or service to the patient. In case management, this means that consent must be obtained from the patient before case management services can be provided. The process to obtain an informed consent may be provided by the facility or organization where the case manager is employed, or may be obtained directly by the case manager. It is the case manager's responsibility to know and follow the process for obtaining informed consent at his or her place of employment.

To carry out the legal steps involved in informed consent, the following requirements must be met when obtaining it from a patient or family member:

- ► *Capacity:* Ensuring that the person consenting is competent and of legal age to consent
- ► *Voluntariness:* Ensuring that the person consenting is exercising freedom of choice without force, fraud, deceit, duress, or coercion
- ► *Information:* Ensuring that the information provided is understandable by the person consenting

The patient bill of rights adopted by most institutions requires the disclosure of the following elements to be considered informed consent:

- ► Diagnosis
- ► Proposed treatment and probability of success
- ► Substantial risks and benefits of the proposed treatment
- ► Alternatives to the proposed treatment
- ► Substantial risks and benefits of alternative treatments

In addition to the above steps, informed consent means that the healthcare professional answers any questions the patient may have and allows the patient to withdraw consent at any time. The informed consent should be witnessed by a second objective person who can attest to the fact that the patient is informed.

Informed consent is either actual or implied. Actual consent means that the healthcare professional has explained the risks, the alternative procedures, and the expected consequences to the appropriate person, and has received a signed consent. Implied consent is common in an emergency situation when an ill or injured person is unable to grant actual consent. Implied consent allows paramedics and emergency medical technicians (EMTs) to transport a person to a healthcare facility for treatment in an emergency situation without the patient's written consent. A situation is generally considered an emergency when a patient is suffering from a life-threatening disease or injury that requires immediate treatment (Romano, 1996). Implied consent is also applied in an emergency situation when a minor child requires medical treatment and a parent's consent cannot be obtained.

Shared Medical Decision-Making — Informed Decision-Making

Shared medical decision-making is a process by which patients and providers consider outcome probabilities and patient preferences and reach a healthcare decision based on mutual agreement. Shared decision-making is best used for problems involving medical uncertainty. During the process, the provider-patient dyad considers treatment options and consequences and explores the fit of expected benefits and consequences of treatment with patient preferences for various outcomes (Frosch, 1999).

Guardianship

The purpose of guardianship is to promote the general welfare of persons who are incapacitated. Guardianship is a legal relationship, appointed by the court, between one person (the guardian) and an incapacitated party. The guardian has the duty and the right to act on behalf of the incapacitated party to make decisions regarding the incapacitated person's life. Unless the guardian is limited by the court in his or her duties, management of all the personal, legal, and financial affairs of the incapacitated person is expected.

In general, guardianship is classified in two categories, known as guardianship of person and guardianship of trust. Establishing guardianship is a means of establishing a legal system that provides incapacitated persons with the rights to:

- ▶ Participate as fully as possible in all decisions that affect them
- ▶ Achieve essential and ongoing physical health and safety
- ▶ Manage their financial resources
- ▶ Develop or regain their abilities to the maximum extent possible
- ▶ Accomplish the aforementioned objectives in the least restrictive environment and through the least restrictive alternatives

The appointed guardian can be a family member, such as a spouse or parent. When a family member is appointed, it is often the next of kin. When a family member or next of kin is not able or willing to serve as guardian, or when the court determines that a family member is not the best choice for an incapacitated person, the appointed guardian may be a professional guardian known to the court and trained in guardianship.

A *guardian ad litem* is a guardian appointed to represent a child. This is necessary when there is a conflict between the parent(s) and the child or when there is no one who can adequately represent the best interests of the child. This can occur in child abuse cases or in other estranged domestic proceedings, such as custody and visitation proceedings. This also occurs when the parents are deceased or incapacitated. The guardian ad litem has a duty to legally advocate for the child's best interests, which may include access to appropriate health care, special education, or even legal defense. The guardian ad litem can be an attorney appointed by the court, the next of kin, or a professional guardian.

Civil Laws

There are several categories of civil laws: intentional torts, quasi-intentional torts, and unintentional torts. Following are examples of torts that could apply to the practice of nursing.

An *intentional tort* is an act in which the outcome was planned, although the person may not have expected the outcome to harm the other person.

- ▶ *Assault:* To threaten or attempt to touch a person without consent. For example, a patient's orders call for intramuscular injection of a certain medication. The patient refuses to be given the injection and the nurse tells the patient she is going to give the shot anyway.

- ▶ *Battery:* To touch without consent, for example, treating without consent

- ▶ *False imprisonment:* The unwarranted use of restraints or restrictions, for example, restraining a person who is acting against medical advice

Quasi-Intentional Tort

An injury to the economics and dignity of a person is *quasi-intentional tort.* Two types of quasi-intentional torts exist.

- ▶ *Invasion of privacy:* Breach of confidentiality, for example, photographing patients without their consent

- ▶ *Defamation of character:* Slander or libel. Some examples include talking about a patient to another healthcare provider in the elevator while other people are present, disclosing patient information over the telephone, and telling stories about a coworker.

Unintentional Torts

Unintentional torts are acts in which the negative outcome was not intended to happen. These torts are perhaps the most familiar to nurse case managers: negligence and malpractice. The two terms are used interchangeably.

- ▶ *Negligence:* The failure to act as a reasonable and prudent person would have acted in a specific situation. This can apply to nonprofessionals.

- ▶ *Malpractice:* The failure of a professional to use such care as a reasonable and prudent member of the profession would use under similar circumstances, which leads to harm

Reasonable and prudent generally mean the average judgment, foresight, intelligence, and skill that would be expected of a person with similar training and experience. Therefore, nurses can be held both negligent and guilty of malpractice.

In order to prove that malpractice or negligence has occurred, four elements must be established: duty, breach of duty, causation, and damages.

Case Simulation—Negligence: A cable company repairman leaving your home after his work is complete trips on the broken wooden plank of your steps. He breaks his nose when landing on his face on your sidewalk. You are liable for this injury because you failed to repair the steps, provide a warning sign to indicate the problem, and so forth.

Case Simulation—Malpractice: A nurse case manager administering medications gives the patient in room 303 the medications that were on the medication order of the patient in room 302. She fails to double-check the room number, the patient's name, or his ID bracelet. After administering the wrong medication to the wrong patient, the nurse continues on her rounds. The patient in room 303 is allergic to one of the medicines she just administered, goes into shock, has to be coded, becomes vent-dependent, and is now on a ventilator for the rest of his life. This nurse was found guilty of malpractice because the following four circumstances were present and proven in a court of law:

1. Harm occurred to the individual.
2. The nurse was in a situation where she had a duty toward the person harmed.
3. The nurse was found to have failed to fulfill her duty.
4. The harm was shown to have been caused by the breach of duty.

The nurse was legally liable, or accountable, for the outcome, whether intended or unintended, and is subject to punishment.

Remember, whenever discussing legal issues in nursing, it is imperative to review your state's Nurse Practice Act (Medi-Smart, 2012a).

CONFIDENTIALITY

Confidentiality and the issues of confidentiality in health care are far-reaching, diverse, and complex. Confidentiality is protected by federal law under the Healthcare Insurance Portability and Accountability Act (HIPAA), described previously, and under accreditation mandates by The Joint Commission (now the Joint Commission on Accreditation of Healthcare Organizations). In 1988, The Joint Commission identified privacy and confidentiality as two patient rights. Additionally, many case managers are governed ethically to maintain patient confidentiality through their individual licensures and practice acts. The ANA's *Standards of Clinical Nursing Practice* requires the nurse to maintain patient confidentiality. According to ANA's Code of Ethics for Nurses, "It is important for the case manager to understand and adhere to local, state, and federal laws as well as employer policies governing client and patient privacy and confidentiality rights, and to act in a manner consistent with the patient's best interest" (ANA, 2010).

Rather than provide clear-cut answers about how and when to divulge information, these authorities can sometimes cause greater confusion for the case manager. In the collaborative role, the case manager is responsible for discussing a patient's condition, prognosis, and other confidential information with many different healthcare professionals and players—physicians, nurses, therapists, social services representatives, insurance company utilization review (UR) nurses and case managers, medical coding and billing personnel, risk managers and quality improvement professionals, claims adjusters, attorneys, and the patient's family or caregiver. In view of the many restrictions placed on confidentiality, it is a good rule of thumb for the case manager to reveal and discuss only the information that is essential for the other party to know—that which is in the best interest of the patient.

Special circumstances, diagnoses, and conditions are governed under various states' legislation, which further convolutes the rules regarding patient confidentiality. Examples include medical records of patients seeking treatment in drug and alcohol abuse rehabilitation programs, and records of HIV-positive patients. Most states have some degree of confidentiality for individuals with HIV-positive test results, including mandates for disclosure of HIV information, and for obtaining consent for testing procedures.

Many cases brought to litigation in the malpractice arena hinge on documentation or the lack of it, resulting in poor communication between healthcare providers of the same and different disciplines. Hand-offs to subsequent caretakers for continuation of care are of particular concern. The first thing a nurse should be aware of is who will be reading the document and why, including: members of the healthcare team, the nurse for her or his own purposes, lawyers and experts, and judge and jury.

DOCUMENTATION

Documentation by the nurse case manager is more important today than ever before because of the variety of providers who see the patient, the variety of settings in which patients receive care, and the many transitions during which care occurs. Appropriate, accurate, and timely documentation is pivotal to protecting the patient's interest as well as the case manager's. Many malpractice cases have revolved around documentation. Case managers are well aware of the adage, "If you didn't document it, it wasn't done," and it still holds true today in court. Good documentation will help you defend yourself in a malpractice lawsuit; it can also keep you out of court in the first place. However, the type of nursing information that appears in a patient's medical record isn't dictated by the courts, but by standards set by the profession, as well as state legislators and regulators. Professional organizations, such as the ANA, and accrediting bodies, such as The Joint Commission and the Centers for Medicare and Medicaid Services (CMS), have established that documentation must include ongoing assessment, variations from assessment, patient teaching, responses to therapies and treatments, and relevant patient statements (Medi-Smart, 2012b).

Documentation continues to be the thread that connects all of the complex processes of patient care coordination in all healthcare settings. This responsibility is personified when the healthcare professional is the case manager, because the case manager is responsible for overall care coordination. If the case manager's involvement in a patient's care includes required compliance with state or federal law, the case manager should also document that the work was conducted within the guidelines of federal or state law. Documentation by the case manager is critical to provide a fluid picture of the patient's journey through the continuum of care. Documented information should be objective—free of suspicion, conjecture, and allegations—because these documents are legally discoverable and can be subpoenaed.

When working with providers, the case manager should require all providers to submit documentation on a periodic basis. The documentation should be clear and concise, and should detail the provider's plan of care, the patient's response to the plan of care, the patient's understanding of the plan of care, and the goals that are being met. Pertinent information should be shared with the treating physician to assist him or her in determining further treatment, as well as recognizing the ability of the patient to assume normal or modified activities, such as a return to work.

Payer-based case managers document their activities and incorporate providers' documentation within the patient care plan. The care plan is available to identified authorities within the payer organization, as well as to the treating physician and other members of the healthcare team when appropriate. The care plan must also be available to the patient upon request (see the section on confidentiality earlier in this chapter) or the patient's attorney, if any. Provider-based case managers submit their documentation to identified authorities within the provider organization, along with the payer case manager, the treating physician when appropriate, other members of the healthcare team when appropriate, and the patient or the patient's attorney.

Case Simulation: In 1997, a case from the Court of Appeals of Georgia pointed out the legal importance of accurate and thorough nursing documentation. The following is a summary of an actual court case, Brown vs. DeKalb Medical Center, 482 S.E. 2d 511 (Ga. App., 1997).

Elderly patients with poor circulation are at high risk for developing pressure sores. When a patient at risk for pressure sores is discharged from nursing care, the heels, buttocks, and other areas should be examined carefully. A nursing note should be made whether or not pressure sores are found.

The court's ruling came in a civil professional negligence lawsuit against a hospital's skilled nursing facility, filed by the family of a now-deceased patient who had undergone a below-the-knee amputation of her left leg for a problem, which allegedly originated as a pressure sore on her heel.

The patient had an area of redness on her sacrum when she came to the nursing facility. It was carefully examined and documented in the acute care nursing notes when the patient was transferred to skilled nursing care, and it was carefully documented again when the patient was sent home after a month in the skilled nursing unit. As to the patient's sacrum, none of the expert witnesses called to testify on either side of the lawsuit could say that this bedsore was any worse when the patient left the skilled nursing unit than when she came in. The court concluded from the nursing documentation of the sacral area that there was no nursing negligence in the care given to this area of the patient's body, and no damages were awarded to the family.

However, there was no documentation one way or the other about the condition of the patient's heels when she was discharged from skilled nursing care. A home health nurse found a fairly fresh lesion on the left heel, which she would later testify could have arisen in the skilled nursing facility before discharge or could have started after the patient got home. The court did not accept at face value the testimony of the nurses from the skilled nursing facility. They said it was their practice not to document a pressure sore on a particular area of a patient's body when none existed.

To satisfy the court and protect themselves from legal liability, the nurses should have entered positive nursing documentation in the chart that the heels had been inspected and that no evidence of a pressure sore could be found. The absence of documentation of a pressure sore on the heel was not the same as positive documentation that none existed, the court said.

The court approved the facility's practices for padding and elevating patients' feet and turning patients every 2 hours, but general statements about routine nursing practices were not enough to avoid liability in this case (Medi-Smart, 1997).

Remember, nurses should document based on evidence-based practice and the standards of care of a reasonable and prudent nurse.

Delegation of Care

- ▶ A contractual agreement in which authority and responsibility for a task is transferred by the person accountable for the task to another person

- ▶ When performed appropriately, delegation benefits the delegator, the delegatee, the organization, and the patient

- ▶ Effective and appropriate delegation minimizes the risk of error, injury, and liability

CONFLICT OF INTEREST

If a public official or fiduciary who, contrary to the obligation and absolute duty to act for the benefit of the public or a designated person, exploits the relationship for personal benefit, typically pecuniary, it is a *conflict of interest.*

In certain relationships, individuals or the general public place their trust and confidence in someone to act in their best interests. When a person has the responsibility to represent another person—whether as administrator, attorney, executor, government official, or trustee—a clash between professional obligations and personal interests arises if the person tries to perform that duty while at the same time trying to achieve personal gain. The appearance of a conflict of interest is present if there is a potential for the personal interests of a person to clash with fiduciary duties, such as when a client has his or her attorney commence an action against a company in which the attorney is the majority stockholder.

Incompatibility of professional duties and personal interests has led Congress and many state legislatures to enact statutes defining conduct that constitutes a conflict of interest and specifying the sanctions for violations. A member of a profession who has been involved in a conflict of interest might be subject to disciplinary proceedings before the body that granted permission to practice that profession

However, conflicts of interest do not apply only to professionals. A conflict of interest arises when anyone has two duties that conflict. When the private interest comes into conflict with the official duty of the person, the conflict can potentially interfere with objective professional judgment. Conflict of interest can be actual, apparent, or potential. In an apparent conflict of interest, a reasonable person can believe that the professional's judgment is likely to be compromised. A potential conflict of interest is one that may develop into an actual conflict of interest, and an actual conflict of interest is when the conflict does occur.

In the role of the case manager, there are many opportunities to unintentionally engage in apparent, potential, or actual conflict of interest.

Case Simulation: A case manager works in an acute care hospital where a manufacturing representative for glucose monitors often visits to introduce staff members to equipment available for patients. Although the case manager does not directly purchase the equipment, the representative recognizes her ability to educate and influence patients' decisions about equipment. Because of her acquaintance with the representative, she can secure a summer job for her daughter with the representative's company. In return, she has a conversation with the hospital's purchasing office and asks that the hospital consider using this aforementioned company's glucose monitors exclusively.

Obviously, conflict of interest often can and does occur in health care. In order to avoid conflict of interest, the case manager should continually consider whether the situation is likely to interfere or appear to interfere with independent, objective judgment. If this is not clear, consider whether trust would be compromised if other people knew of the situation. There are multiple ways to manage conflict of interest. One is to avoid the conflict altogether. Another is to disclose the perceived, potential, or actual conflict of interest to the appropriate parties before participating in the action. Another is to abstain from any decision-making associated with the private interest.

Usually, it is easier to recognize conflict of interest in someone else than in oneself. Personal interests cloud objectivity, or the person may believe he or she can always separate private interest from official duty, thus failing to critically analyze potential conflict of interest before it arises. A good practice is to follow this metaphor: Pass the situation into your mind, where you analyze it, and out of your heart, where you feel it. If it still seems right, it probably is.

ACCESS TO CARE

One of the most pressing legal and ethical problems nurse case managers and all people in the United States face today is access to care. Many factors, such as culture, economics, legislation, and politics affect access to care. After all, all health care is local and all politics is local. In the United States, the greatest barrier to accessing health care is insurance—or the lack thereof. According to the Census Bureau data on health insurance coverage and the uninsured for 2010, the percentage of people without health insurance in 2010 was 16.3%, approximately 50 million people. Nine in 10 of the uninsured are in low- or moderate-income families, meaning they are below 400% of poverty. Young adults are the age group least likely to have health insurance. The percentage of children under age 18 without health insurance in 2010 was 9.8%. Employer-sponsored insurance continued to be the largest source of health insurance coverage in 2010, covering 55.3% of the population. However, according to the Kaiser Commission, more than three quarters of the uninsured are in working families. Because the average annual cost of employer-sponsored family coverage in 2010 is $13,770, many cannot afford the premiums without sizable employer contributions (Kaiser, 2011). Uninsured rates for Hispanics (30.7%) and Blacks (20.8%) are higher than for non-Hispanic Whites (11.7%).

Health insurance in the United States is provided through several major private and public sources. For calendar year 2010:

▶ 55.3% of the population was covered by employer-sponsored insurance

▶ 14.5% of the population was covered by Medicare and 15.9% was covered by Medicaid — with some people covered by both programs

▶ 4.2% of the population was covered by military health services

▶ 16.3% of the population was uninsured for the entire year (U.S. Department of Health and Human Services, 2011)

However, even when patients have insurance, the nurse case manager is faced with the challenge of understanding and assisting patients in understanding their insurance benefit packages, such as which services are covered, which providers are in the network, what the copays are, and so on. The case manager must use his or her skills in resource management to find entities that may cover the needed services if they are not covered in the patient's benefit package. Whether or not services are covered, case managers have an ethical responsibility to provide whatever services are possible that are in the best interest of the patient.

Insurance is not the only barrier to accessing health care, however. The system itself presents challenges to those who try to navigate through it.

▶ Language: Many people are forced to seek care from providers who do not speak their language.

▶ Site availability: Many healthcare sites are great distances from people's homes, or the sites are not open during hours that are convenient for them. For example, health centers often are not open after 5 p.m. or on Saturdays.

Additionally, the so-called system in place for people to enroll in government-sponsored insurance programs is cumbersome, time-consuming, unclear, and difficult to find.

Many states and accrediting bodies have "access to care" standards by which providers and health plan networks must abide. These standards address not only access to care, but also timely access to care. The standards cover the time frames in which a patient must be seen in an emergency situation, an urgent situation, and when he or she seeks routine care. Access and availability studies are routinely conducted and providers are penalized for nonadherence.

Sometimes, access to care is not achieved because the patient refuses the care that is available or offered. This situation is especially frustrating for the case manager accustomed to working diligently to access appropriate services. However, a patient's right to self-determination dictates that the patient can refuse access to available care. Before accepting a patient's refusal of care, the case manager should ensure that the patient has received adequate information to make an informed decision. If a patient has received adequate information, is able to make an informed decision, and still refuses care, the case manager should document this activity, including the information about the expected outcomes both with and without the service, and that the patient has refused the service.

Cost vs. Quality

Quality, cost, service—pick any two. It sounds silly, but today's nurse case managers are faced with just these types of decisions. If you want high-quality care delivered by a top-performing provider at a premier healthcare facility, you will not get it at a low cost. If low cost is what a nurse case manager is looking for, he or she probably will not get high-quality care and a top-performing provider to deliver that care at a premier site. However, when considering quality versus cost, reimbursement should not be the primary consideration for the nurse case manager, and he or she should always err on the side of quality.

During the early 1990s, managed care began to proliferate in the healthcare arena. This acceleration of managed care penetration posed new challenges for nurse case managers and all providers. Managed care was becoming deeply entrenched in the fiber of the commercial insurance industry and was now making deeper inroads in the government-sponsored insurance programs. Several states were mandating enrollment in managed care organizations (MCOs) for their Medicaid enrollees. Many felt this "gatekeeper" model was designed to keep costs down while limiting access to high-quality healthcare services. In order to safeguard people against any negative impact on their health care, a Health Care Bill of Rights that required managed care plans to meet specific standards of operation was passed. The bill contained essential consumer protections to ensure access to care and confidentiality of medical records. It also contained provisions for enrollee outreach, continuity of care, provider choice, and a system for reporting data collected by the plan.

Shortly following this legislation, the NCQA was formed. This organization brought together experts in all fields of health care and developed a set of criteria by which managed care organizations would be measured. These measures are now called the Healthcare Effectiveness Data and Information Set (HEDIS). These measures looked at all aspects of the managed care business—access to care, utilization of services, stability of the plan, strength of the provider network, and quality of care. (NCQA and HEDIS are discussed in detail in Chapter 4.) Today there are national benchmarks by which plans are measured.

The quality versus cost discussion was not limited to MCOs. The Institute of Medicine (IOM), in its reports, looked at the quality and cost of health care being delivered in hospitals. Additionally, professional organizations were looking at how practitioners were measuring up to the standards of care endorsed by their peer organizations. Accreditation for institutions, MCOs, and healthcare vendors, and certification for providers, also gave weight to the positive side of the ledger in the quality versus cost debate.

Other quality versus costs concerns were raised in the 1980s and 1990s when two new payment systems came into play—diagnostic-related groups (DRGs) and capitation. DRGs were payment rates assigned to specific diagnostic codes. If a case manager's patient was admitted into the hospital with a certain diagnosis, the hospital was reimbursed the same amount of money if the patient stayed in the facility for 2 days or 20 days. Obviously, the perceived or real push then became to get patients through the system, procedures, and services as quickly as possible and discharged as early as possible so the institution could remain viable. At the time, the buzz was that patients were discharged "quicker and sicker."

The other reimbursement system that caused some concern was capitation. This system was counterintuitive to the way the fee-for-service model had been operating. In fee for service, patients pay for the services they receive as they receive them. This capitation model was designed to pay providers the same amount of money monthly for every member on their roster, whether they were seen once or a dozen times in that month. The fear here was that providers would not reach out to those members who were not seeking care because they were being paid for them already, whether they saw them or not. Quality measures were introduced to address the impact of both of these reimbursement systems. For example, readmission rates—were patients being discharged and then readmitted within the next 30 days? Today if that occurs for certain diagnoses, the hospitals are denied payment. An example of quality measures designed to keep the capitation model functioning well are HEDIS measures that look at utilization of services and preventive care services delivered.

As time marches forward, so do ideas for different payment methodologies. Therefore, it was no surprise to see the next generation of methodologies, called CRGs, developed by 3M. These Clinical Risk Groups (CRGs) provide a means of adjusting payment amounts according to the clinical characteristics and resource demands of patients. Although DRGs and 3M Clinical Risk Groups are both classification systems, DRGs measure inpatient resource utilization, while 3M CRGS capture the resource utilization of all inpatient and ambulatory encounters during a chosen time period (usually a year). In addition, yet another reimbursement methodology appeared, All Patient Refined DRGs, which classify acute care patients and are specifically designed to adjust data for severity of illness and risk of mortality.

Another view of quality versus cost comes through the pay-for-performance lens, discussed in Chapter 4. This new phenomenon reimburses providers more money for delivering high-quality care. This, of course, raises the question: Why aren't practitioners delivering high-quality care to begin with? That brings us to the next topic in this chapter, ethics.

ETHICS

> **"**Ethics is knowing the difference between what you have a right to do and what is right to do.**"**
> —*Potter Stewart*

Nurse case managers are constantly challenged to make ethical decisions while serving their patients. Their roles as negotiators, educators, and advocates may at times be at odds with one another. For example, as negotiator, the case manager may negotiate with the patient about adherence to a care plan. In this instance, when the case manager is discussing a behavioral change, he or she must be aware that the discussion is usually governed by personal values on both sides, and sometimes the case manager's values are a strong determining factor. It is important that the case manager understand the principles of ethics and what steps he or she can take to safeguard against crossing that imaginary ethical line.

In today's healthcare arena, the nurse case manager is challenged every day with making decisions that involve balancing quality of care and cost. These challenges may come from patients, providers, advocates, communities, society in general, or a combination of these, and take many different forms. At times, nurse case managers are challenged by the patient who is refusing services or refusing to change harmful behaviors. Some case managers are challenged by providers who are inaccessible, by insurance benefit packages that are inadequate to meet the needs of their patients, or by services that are needed but are not authorized by an insurance carrier. Therefore, the nurse case manager must have a working understanding of the Code of Ethics set by the American Nurses Association and the ethical principles set forth in the CMSA's *Standards of Practice*.

Over the years, the Nursing Code of Ethics has evolved. It began in 1893 with the Nightingale Pledge:

> *I solemnly pledge myself before God and in the presence of this assembly, to pass my life in purity and to practice my profession faithfully. I will abstain from whatever is deleterious and mischievous, and will not take or knowingly administer any harmful drug. I will do all in my power to maintain and elevate the standard of my profession, and will hold in confidence all personal matters committed to my keeping and all family affairs coming to my knowledge in the practice of my calling. With loyalty will I endeavor to aid the physician, in his work, and devote myself to the welfare of those committed to my care.* (ANA, 2008)

Today, the Nightingale pledge is not the ANA's Code of Ethics, but the overarching message has remained the same as seen in this statement: "The nurse's role in Ethics and Human Rights: Protecting and promoting individual worth, dignity, and human rights in practice settings. Respect for the inherent dignity, worth, and uniqueness of every individual, is a fundamental principle that underlies all nursing practice" (ANA, 2010a).

This Code of Ethics makes explicit the primary goals, values, and obligations of the profession. It serves as a succinct statement of the nonnegotiable ethical obligations and duties of every person who enters the nursing profession and the understanding of his or her commitment to society. It has nine provisions that describe the most fundamental values and commitments of the nurse, and addresses boundaries of duty and loyalty and aspects of duty beyond the individual patient encounters.

CMSA's Standard: Ethics

Case managers should behave and practice ethically, adhering to the tenets of the code of ethics that underlies his or her professional credential (e.g., nursing, social work, rehabilitation counseling, etc.). How Demonstrated: Awareness of the five basic ethical principles and how they are applied: beneficence (to do good), nonmalfeasance (to do no harm), autonomy (to respect individuals' rights to make their own decisions), justice (to treat others fairly), and fidelity (to follow-through and to keep promises). Recognition that a case manager's primary obligation is to his/her clients. Maintenance of respectful relationships with coworkers, employers, and other professionals. Recognition that laws, rules, policies, insurance benefits, and regulations are sometimes in conflict with ethical principles. In such situations, case managers are bound to address such conflicts to the best of their abilities and/or seek appropriate consultation. (CMSA, 2010, p. 19)

ETHICAL PRINCIPLES

Ethical principles serve as guidelines for case managers in their daily practice. These include the five moral principles of autonomy, beneficence, nonmaleficence, justice, and veracity. Each case manager is responsible for understanding the obligations and duties of a case manager, and for incorporating moral principles into daily practice. To accomplish this, case managers in every job setting should objectively judge their ability to practice ethically in their employment (Tillman, 1994). One way to accomplish this is to consider the following questions:

▶ What is expected of me as an employee?

▶ Is my job description in conflict with my own moral beliefs?

▶ Am I expected to make compromises in the best interest of my employer, and if so, are there alternatives if these decisions compromise my ethical practice?

▶ Is cost containment the bottom line, and if so, to what extent am I expected to control costs?

▶ Are there processes in place to make exceptions for patients who need services or products that may cost more money?

▶ Are there processes in place for objective decisions to be made regarding patient care?

▶ Is quality measured by the employer, and are there written policies and procedures in place for continuous quality improvement?

▶ Will I be provided with opportunities for continuing education to advance my professional knowledge in the field?

The case manager should always have the ability to practice ethically in the employment setting. Moral principles must be applied to the case manager's daily practice.

Autonomy

Autonomy is the moral principle governing a person's right to make his or her own decisions. It is respect for others and for their uniqueness. In health care, the patient should be encouraged to make decisions about his or her healthcare treatment, even if the decisions are difficult for healthcare providers to accept. The principle of autonomy is evident in the Patient Self-Determination Act of 1990, a law, discussed earlier in this chapter, that was prompted by a patient's need to determine in advance whether he or she desires life-supporting measures should he or she become incapacitated by injury or illness. Autonomy promotes independence and gives the patient an inherent right to determine what happens according to his or her own preferences and value system.

Beneficence

Beneficence is the moral principle governing a person's obligation to promote good, to further a person's legitimate interests, and to actively prevent or remove harm. Beneficence requires the case manager to promote the well-being of the patient and family within the constraints of the healthcare system. This includes using good resource management skills to promote a safe discharge for the patient. If an elderly female patient with a fractured hip has no one at home to assist her with activities of daily living, for example, the patient is at risk of falling and is an unsafe discharge. A wheelchair-bound patient cannot safely be discharged to a home environment that has steps and narrow doorways.

Nonmaleficence

Nonmaleficence means to refrain from doing harm to others. Case managers can gauge nonmaleficence by understanding and incorporating outcome measurements into their daily practices. Outcomes can provide a picture of the quality, cost, and appropriateness of care delivered to a patient. Information on outcome measurements is covered in Chapter 4. More formal methods of governing nonmaleficence are provided through ethics committees established in many healthcare settings. Ethics committees are intended to provide objective means to promote nonmaleficence and other forms of ethical practice. Ethics committees are particularly active in acute care settings, where ethical dilemmas often arise surrounding such issues as high-tech medical care, advance directives, conflicting wishes of family members, mental competence of patients, surrogacy, and unsafe discharges or transfers.

Justice

Justice is defined as maintaining what is right and fair. It is the moral principle that governs the responsibility of the case manager to coordinate the appropriate allocation of resources to meet the patient's healthcare needs. It is a moral principle that, when practiced consistently, can establish and promote trust between the patient and the case manager. Case managers should also practice justice when collaborating with other members of the healthcare team, including payers and providers. If a case manager considers what is right and fair before making decisions and recommendations about healthcare services and resources, he or she is practicing the golden rule—doing unto others as you would have them do unto you. This will clearly promote trust from others about the actions and intent of the case manager.

Veracity

Veracity is truth-telling, and it also is an important component of developing a trusting relationship with the patient, family, providers, and payers. In today's healthcare climate, there exists an unfortunate element of mistrust among many patients, who are put off by a convoluted healthcare delivery system. Further, physicians often mistrust payers. Healthcare professionals often mistrust one another's actions. Overall, it is sometimes a difficult climate in which to promote trust-building for the patient, who is most vulnerable during illness or injury. Veracity can promote trust and enhance trusting relationships.

Patient's Bill of Rights

Below is a summary of a bill of rights that was adopted by the U.S. President's Advisory Commission on in 1998. This bill of rights now applies to the insurance plans offered to federal employees. Many other health plans and facilities have also adopted these values. Even Medicare and Medicaid stand by many of them. In addition to this bill of rights focused on hospitals and insurance plans, there are many other versions. There are special kinds, such as the mental health bill of rights, hospice patient's bill of rights, and bills of rights for patients in certain states. Insurance plans sometimes have lists of rights for subscribers. Many of these documents tell patients where to go or whom to talk with if they have a problem with their care. The following are the American Hospital Association list of rights, along with patient responsibilities that can help a person be a more active partner in his or her health care.

Information disclosure: You have the right to accurate and easily understood information about your health plan, healthcare professionals, and healthcare facilities. If you speak another language, have a physical or mental disability, or just don't understand something, help should be provided so you can make informed healthcare decisions.

Choice of providers and plans: You have the right to a choice of healthcare providers who can give you high-quality health care when you need it.

Access to emergency services: If you have severe pain, an injury, or sudden illness that makes you believe that your health is in serious danger, you have the right to be screened and stabilized using emergency services. These services should be provided whenever and wherever you need them, without the need to wait for authorization and without any financial penalty.

Participation in treatment decisions: You have the right to know your treatment options and to take part in decisions about your care. Parents, guardians, family members, or others who you select can represent you if you cannot make your own decisions.

Respect and nondiscrimination: You have a right to considerate, respectful care from your doctors, health plan representatives, and other healthcare providers that does not discriminate against you.

Confidentiality of health information: You have the right to talk privately with healthcare providers and to have your healthcare information protected. You also have the right to read and copy your own medical record. You have the right to ask that your doctor change your record if it is not accurate, relevant, or complete.

Complaints and appeals: You have the right to a fair, fast, and objective review of any complaint you have against your health plan, doctors, hospitals, or other healthcare personnel. This includes complaints about waiting times, operating hours, the actions of healthcare personnel, and the adequacy of healthcare facilities (American Cancer Society, 2010).

On November 5, 1990, Congress passed the Patient Self-Determination Act (PSDA) as an amendment to the Omnibus Budget Reconciliation Act of 1990. It became effective on December 1, 1991. The PSDA requires many Medicare and Medicaid providers (hospitals, nursing homes, hospice programs, home health agencies, and HMOs) to give adults, at the time of inpatient admission or enrollment, certain information about their rights under state laws governing advance directives, including

▶ The right to participate in and direct their own healthcare decisions
▶ The right to accept or refuse medical or surgical treatment
▶ The right to prepare an advance directive
▶ The right to information on the provider's policies that govern the use of these rights

The act also prohibits institutions from discriminating against a patient who does not have an advance directive. The PSDA further requires institutions to document patient information and provide ongoing community education on advance directives (Ascension Health, 2007).

ADVANCE DIRECTIVES

Advance directives are written documents in which people specify what type of medical care they want in the future should they lose their ability to make decisions. The decision to have an advance directive is purely voluntary. No family member, hospital, or insurance company can force someone to have one, or dictate what the document should say. There are two types of advance directives: a durable power of attorney for health care and a living will. A durable power of attorney for health care, also known as a healthcare proxy, is a document that grants another person power to make medical treatment and related personal care decisions on his or her behalf. In most states it is legally binding.

A living will is a written statement in which a person informs doctors and family members what types of medical care he or she wishes to receive should he or she become terminally ill or permanently unconscious, and unable to make or communicate decisions about continued care.

There are differences between a durable power of attorney for health care and a living will. The focus of a durable power of attorney for health care is on who makes the decision, while the focus of a living will is on what the decisions are. Furthermore, a living will is limited to care during terminal illness or permanent unconsciousness, while a durable power of attorney for health care can be applicable during temporary disability.

An example of a patient's intent to direct and control the degree of medical treatment administered is a "do not resuscitate" order, also know as a DNR. Case managers are responsible for being familiar with the scope of the law on advance directives in states where they practice, because healthcare professionals are responsible for implementing advance directives on the patient's behalf. Advance directives are intended to remove all questions and doubts from family members and healthcare practitioners regarding the treatment wishes of the individual. Most advance directives allow a person to designate another person to serve as his or her healthcare representative or healthcare surrogate in the event he or she becomes incompetent.

Case managers embedded in facilities should understand their role in securing advance directives and have a working knowledge of their facility's policies and procedures for securing same. Case managers should review patients' charts for the existence of advanced directives and document their existence. Any discussion with the patient regarding an advance directive should be documented. If the patient wishes to rescind the advance directive, the case manager must report this information to the proper authorities identified in the facility's policy and procedures.

As providers continue to be squeezed between mandated services and limited direct patient care, hands-on time and low reimbursement rates, quality of care remains a paramount issue for everyone—nurse case managers, other providers, and the public. Therefore, nurse case managers must continue to look for ways to get patients and the general populace to accept responsibility and become partners in their own health care. It is the only way the case management profession is going to make a difference.

REFERENCES

American Cancer Society. (2010). *The Patient's Bill of Rights.* Retrieved from http://www.cancer.org/Treatment/ FindingandPayingforTreatment/UnderstandingFinancialandLegalMatters/patients-bill-of-rights

American Nurses Association. (2008). *The Florence Nightingale Pledge.* Retrieved from http:// www.nursingworld.org/FunctionalMenuCategories/AboutANA/WhereWeComeFrom_1/ FlorenceNightingalePledge.aspx

American Nurses Association. (2010a). *Code of Ethics for Nurses with interpretive statements.* Silver Spring, MD: Author. Available at http://www.nursingworld.org/MainMenuCategories/EthicsStandards/ CodeofEthicsforNurses/Code-of-Ethics.pdf

American Nurses Association. (2010b). *Nursing's social policy statement: The essence of the profession.* Silver Spring, MD: Author. Available at http://gm6.nursingworld.org/MainMenuCategories/Policy- Advocacy/Positions-and-Resolutions/ANAPositionStatements/Position-Statements-Alphabetically/ Nursess-Role-in-Ethics-and-Human-Rights.pdf

Americans with Disabilities Act of 1990. Pub. L. 101–336, 42 U.S.C. § 12101.

Ascension Health. (2007). *Patient Self-Determination Act.* Retrieved from www.ascensionhealth.org/ethics/ public/issues/patient_self.asp

Case Management Society of America. (2010). *Standards of practice for case management.* Little Rock, AR: Author.

Centers for Medicare and Medicaid Services. (2011). *Medicare managed care manual,* Retrieved from https://www.cms.gov/manuals/iom/itemdetail.asp?itemid=CMS019326

Centers for Medicare and Medicaid Services. (2012). *Overview of prescription drug coverage: General information.* Retrieved from https://www.cms.gov/PrescriptionDrugCovGenIn/

Frosch. D. L., & Kaplan, R. M. (1999). Shared decision making in clinical medicine: Past research and future directions. *American Journal of Preventative Medicine, 17*(4), 285-294.

H.R. 6983—110th Congress: Paul Wellstone and Pete Domenici Mental Health Parity and Addiction Equity Act of 2008. (2008). In GovTrack.us (database of federal legislation). Retrieved from http://www. govtrack.us/congress/bills/110/hr6983

Kaiser. (2011). *Kaiser Commision on Medicaid and the Uninsured: A mid-year state Medicaid budget update for FY 2012 and a look forward to FY 2013 executive summary.* Retrieved from http://www.kff.org/ medicaid/8277.cfm

Medi-Smart. (1997). Pressure sores: Court case points out importance of nursing documentation. *Legal Eagle Eye Newsletter, 5*(6), 1. Retrieved from http://medi-smart.com/pressuresores.htm

Medi-Smart. (2012a). *Nursing legal issues: How to protect yourself.* Retrieved from http://www.medi-smart. com/nursing-articles/nursing-law/legal-issues

Medi-Smart. (2012b). *Nursing legal issues: The do's and don'ts of documentation.* Retrieved from http://www. medi-smart.com/nursing-resources/documentation

Mitchell, E. R. (2007). *Elder abuse basics, part 5: What is abandonment?* Retrieved from http://socialwork. about.com

National Council of State Boards of Nursing. (2011). *Nurse licensure compact administrators.* Retrieved from https://www.ncsbn.org/2011_NLCA_factsheet_students_Rev_Jan_2011.pdf

Patient Self-Determination Act of 1990. Pub. L. 101-508.

Powell, S. (1996). *Nursing case management: A practical guide to success in managed care.* Philadelphia: Lippincott, Williams & Wilkins.

Romano, J. (1996). *Legal rights of the catastrophically ill and injured: A family guide.* Philadelphia: Rosenstein & Romano.

Tillman, V. (1994). Ethics. In R. Howe (Ed.), *Case management for healthcare professionals* (pp. 35–38). Chicago: Precept Press.

U.S. Department of Health and Human Services. (2008). *Overview of the uninsured in the United States: An analysis of the 2005 current population survey.* Retrieved from http://aspe.hhs.gov/health/reports/05/uninsured-cps/

U.S. Department of Health and Human Services. (2011). *Summary of HIPAA privacy rule.* Retrieved from http://www.hhs.gov/ocr/privacy/hipaa/understanding/index.html

U.S. Department of Labor. (2008). *Mental Health Parity Act.* Retrieved from http://www.dol.gov/ebsa/newsroom/fsmhparity.html

CHAPTER 6

PRINCIPLES OF EDUCATION AND LEARNING

> **"**If you tell me, I will listen. If you show me, I will see.
> If you let me experience, I will learn.**"**
> —*Lao Tzu*

Effective education is essential to smooth transitions of care and adherence to self-management by patients, families, and caregivers. Nurse case managers (NCM) must consider the individual learning needs of each patient to communicate essential knowledge. Motivation, willingness to change, and a readiness to learn are assessment items for the nurse case manager as a case management plan is developed. NCMs encounter multiple barriers and opportunities as they educate, so anticipating these possibilities, and offering proactive interventions, will result in successful educational encounters. This chapter discusses teaching and learning principles and explores change theory and readiness to learn, as well as issues with health promotion and illness prevention.

The three key outcomes case managers can claim regardless of setting are patient education and empowerment, effective and efficient care coordination, and adherence to the plan of care. By educating and empowering patients, case managers can achieve wellness even in the face of illness or injury. Effective, efficient, and safe transitions of care provide patients, families, and caregivers with access to the most appropriate resources—those necessary to meet their individual needs. Adherence to the plan of care is an essential outcome case managers achieve by recognizing and addressing barriers to care and proactively monitoring patients to ensure that they are making progress toward the ultimate goal of self-management. To accomplish these goals, case managers must be diligent in their education endeavors. An effective educator is one who successfully helps patients and families learn how to care for themselves, prevent further injury or illness, gain control of their lives when faced with healthcare challenges, and achieve quality of life throughout their life spans.

Case managers engage in wellness education by helping patients identify risky behaviors and make simple behavioral changes that can prevent or limit illness and reduce injury. When chronic illnesses are present, case managers provide disease-specific education geared toward raising awareness and understanding of the conditions so that patients can self-manage. When options for aggressive care become limited, case managers initiate discussions regarding end-of-life care options. Other responsibilities in health education include community resources such as transportation or lodging, and education on benefits or health plan coverage, including copays and out-of-pocket expenses. In addition, information regarding risks and benefits of treatment options as well as second opinions may be necessary. Educating stakeholders is a key element to successful, high-quality outcomes. Nurse case managers employ various creative strategies to share healthcare data across the continuum of care.

As professionals, case managers and other healthcare providers must actively participate in their own continuing education efforts in order to be clinically and professionally competent. Professional development is achieved by reading articles in clinical magazines and journals, participating in research projects or inservice classes offered internally as well as through professional organizations, or enrolling in formal classes or online programs, including webinars, that advance knowledge.

Many states and certifying organizations require that healthcare professionals accumulate a specific number of continuing education hours to maintain their licenses or national certifications. Seeking and maintaining current knowledge is essential for nurse case managers who are providing critical services in a complex healthcare system.

In this chapter, the principles of adult learning are covered. Understanding these principles helps professionals in their own educational efforts, as well as provides insight on teaching others. Since children and adolescents learn differently than adults, it is important to gear educational activities toward the specific audience. Insight into the theories of adult learning is gleaned from Malcolm Knowles, a leader in the field of adult education. Knowles first coined the term *andragogy* in the mid-1960s to describe adult learning. *Pedagogy* describes the science of teaching children; andragogy is the art and science of helping adults learn (Conner, 2004). Knowles identified the following characteristics of adult learners. Case managers should use these as guidelines when designing educational programs for adults.

▶ Adults are autonomous and self-directed. Case managers need to actively involve their patients in the learning process and act as facilitators to guide the process. Obtaining patients' perspectives about what their needs are allows them to learn at their own pace in order to reach their healthcare goals.

▶ Unlike children, adults have a foundation of life experience and knowledge base that includes work-related activities, family responsibilities, and previous education. Understanding how to connect these experiences and knowledge when developing educational activities is essential.

▶ Adults are goal-oriented. Taking time to learn patients' goals and developing programs that help them attain those goals are fundamental to the case management process.

▶ Adult learners are relevancy-oriented; they must see a reason for learning. Adults learn best when they can see how following a plan is applicable to work or other responsibilities that they value.

▶ Adults are practical and focus on what is most useful to them. Case managers who focus learning by designing educational programs that clearly demonstrate how information is useful to the patient have more success than those who design general programs on specific topics.

▶ As do all learners, adults need respect. Acknowledging the wealth of experiences that adults bring is important. Treating adults as equals in experience and knowledge and allowing them to express their opinions are important to the relationship between case managers and patients (Keesee, 2011).

Four critical elements of learning that case managers must understand when developing activities designed to enhance the educational process are:

▶ Motivation

▶ Reinforcement

▶ Retention

▶ Transference (Merriam & Caffarella, 1999)

Motivation

It's important to motivate patients to achieve successful learning. Setting a positive tone for the lesson by establishing a friendly, open atmosphere helps portray the case manager's desire to help the patient. If the patient does not recognize the need for the information or has been offended, experts agree that all efforts to assist the patient in the learning process will be in vain. Establishing rapport with the patient provides the motivation needed to engage him or her.

In addition, most people learn best under low or moderate stress. If a patient's stress level is too high, learning becomes a barrier. Program design should challenge the learner to his or her education level, but not be so high as to cause frustration or information overload.

Copious amounts of healthcare information are available, so it is important to gauge the patient's tolerance for the amount of information he or she can comprehend.

Another important point that case managers as educators should be aware of is the importance of providing feedback to the patient as part of the learning process. Feedback that is specific to the patient is more effective than general feedback. When a patient perceives a reward for his or her efforts, the patient is further motivated. Rewards do not need to be tangible, but can be simply a demonstration of the benefits realized from learning the material.

Reinforcement

Reinforcement is a necessary part of the teaching and learning process. It encourages correct modes of behavior and performance. Two types of reinforcement exist—positive and negative. Positive reinforcement is good; it reinforces positive behavior. Negative reinforcement is useful in trying to change modes of behavior. The result of negative reinforcement occurs when the case manager uses negative reinforcement until the bad behavior disappears. Experts say that when trying to change behavior, both positive and negative reinforcement are necessary. To maintain consistent, positive behavior, reinforcement should be part of the teaching and learning process.

Retention

An essential outcome of the learning process is retention. In order for learners to retain information, they must see its meaning or purpose and how it relates to them. They must also understand how to interpret and apply the information. Experts explain that retention is directly affected by the amount of practice applied during the learning experience. For example, case managers can assess retention by asking patients for a return demonstration to evaluate if the information was learned. This exercise provides an opportunity for the case manager to clarify points and allows time to explain again or clarify parts of the lesson as needed. Taking this extra step as part of the education process ensures the information taught was understood and incorporated as need.

Transference

The transfer of learning with the end result of the training being the ability to use the information taught in a new setting or context is the final critical element of learning. To achieve this, the case manager can ask the patient how he or she can incorporate the information into his or her life. Asking the patient to keep a journal allows both patient and case manager to review the patient's progress and how well he or she incorporated the information into "real-life" situations. This allows the case manager to determine if information needs to be reviewed or to address any challenges the patient may have with an exercise. It also allows the patient to identify and discuss patterns and barriers. As noted previously, this extra step ensures that the information taught can be put into action.

CHANGE THEORY AND CONCEPTS

Nurse case managers have many roles, perhaps none as essential and challenging as that of change agent. Healthcare providers and patients have a shared responsibility for behavior changes that maximize wellness and promote disease prevention. Lifestyle choice and risk behaviors such as smoking, inactivity, unhealthy diets, and nonadherence to medications contribute to an increase in morbidity and mortality, plus escalating healthcare costs.

Multiple theorists have examined motivations to change, behavioral changes, and sustaining change. The Transtheoretical Model of Behavior Change (TTM) describes six stages that people move through to modify behaviors:

- ► Precontemplation
- ► Contemplation
- ► Preparation
- ► Action
- ► Maintenance
- ► Termination

TTM recognizes that change is a process that unfolds over time, involving progress through a series of stages (Prochaska & Prochaska, 2011). Understanding how people change, and the theoretical model behind it, is critical for nurse case managers who serve diverse populations with multiple health issues. Advising patients on the risks of their behaviors, and the consequences of continuing unhealthy choices, is an appropriate case management function.

LEARNER READINESS

Health education and health promotion programs are directly linked to the theories of adult education and, more specifically, to the theories of behavioral change. Knowles, a pioneer in the field of adult education, advocated that education must be learner-centered, built on the needs and interest of learners. More specifically, his model is based on three main assumptions: adults are self-directed learners, adults require a readiness to learn, and their orientation to learning is problem- or life-centered. These assumptions form the basis for many health education and behavioral change programs that case managers use when working with patients. Theorists involved in the study of behavioral change suggest that adults are more likely to adopt healthy practices and behaviors when

- ► They perceive themselves at risk of developing a specific condition
- ► The condition is perceived to be serious, with negative consequences
- ► The risks will be reduced with specific behavior changes
- ► The barriers to behavior change can be overcome or managed (Diniz, Schmidt, & Stothers, 2008)

Case Simulation: When discharging a 60-year-old man with a history of smoking and who suffered a heart attack, the case manager talks to him about the need to stop smoking. He tells the case manager that he will go to the program as he now knows that his smoking is slowly killing him. He shares that his doctor has told him for years that his smoking was causing him harm, but he never believed him. When writing her notes, the case manager reflects back to the conversation and realizes that so many times patients wait for a major event to happen before making positive lifestyle changes.

Influencing or facilitating behavior change is not always easy. Case managers must address a number of other factors, including the patient's readiness to change, the availability of resources where patients can gain help, the patient's support system, and the level of self-help skills that the patient possesses. Taking the time to understand these issues and work toward finding resources that will meet the individual needs of the patient are important tasks that can produce positive outcomes for both the case manager and, more importantly, the patient.

LEARNING STYLES

Different people learn and process information differently. Research shows that the various learning styles fall into general categories: perceptual modality, information processing, and personality patterns. These categories represent ways to focus on the learner.

► *Perpetual modality* refers to the primary ways our bodies take in information. This occurs visually, through our auditory senses, or through the senses of touch and smell.

► *Information processing* distinguishes among the ways we sense, think, solve problems, and remember information. Each patient has a preferred, consistent, and distinct way of perceiving, organizing, and retaining information.

► *Personality patterns* focus on attention, emotion, and values. Studying these differences allows case managers to predict the way patients will react and feel about different situations.

Most people retain a dominant and an auxiliary learning modality. Traditionally, they rely on those modalities to process information at a subconscious level while being consciously aware of their preferred mode. In other words, people access information through all of their senses—visual, auditory, olfactory, gustatory, kinesthetic, tactile—but generally favor one (Churchill, 2007).

The assessment process is a good opportunity for case managers to listen for key words that can help them understand their patients' learning styles. For example, a visual learner may say, "I see your point." An auditory learner may say, "I hear what you are saying." A kinesthetic learner may say, "I feel we're moving in the right direction." Knowing this allows case managers to understand their patients' preferred learning methods and design programs that meet those styles.

When working with someone who is a visual learner, for example, visual aids—pictures, images, charts, graphs, and so on—help them understand ideas and information better than explanations. Auditory learners prefer the spoken message, even their own voice, to process information. They listen and remember things said to them, and may even carry on mental dialogues and determine how to continue by thinking back on the words of others. Others who fall into this category feel the need to "talk it out," and often talk to those around them. Patients like this may prefer support groups to help work out issues by listening to and talking with others. Kinesthetic learners learn best by moving their bodies, activating their muscles as they learn. Tactile learners want to touch things. Those who fall into this category may say, "Enough talking, let's get to work." These types of learners—kinesthetic and tactile—do best with hands-on projects, are compatible learners, and can be grouped together.

Another important point in assessing learning styles is discovering the patient's motivational style. Understanding this can help the NCM design educational activities that keep patients focused and help them find reasons to stay with the plan until goals are achieved. Common motivational learning styles include

▶ Goal-oriented learners who use education to accomplish their objectives,

▶ Activity-oriented learners who take part mainly because of the social contact they can get from the experience, and

▶ Learning-oriented learners who seek knowledge for its own sake (Conner, 2008).

Recognizing the unique motivational styles of patients can help the NCM identify the types of educational programs that will be most successful. Remember, people can be invited to learn but the motivation must be theirs.

HEALTH LITERACY

The Institute of Medicine addressed this issue in its report *Health Literacy: A Prescription to End Confusion*. In the report, it was noted that 90 million people in the United States have difficulty understanding and using health information. Interacting with the healthcare system, choosing a healthy lifestyle, and seeking appropriate medical care all require using health information. The ability to obtain, process, and understand health information needed to make informed health decisions is known as *health literacy*. Limited health literacy is related to poor health outcomes such as increased hospital admissions, skipping preventive health measures, and increased utilization of heathcare services (U.S. Department of Health and Human Services, 2010). Reasons for limited health literacy include lack of education, limited English proficiency, learning disabilities, cultural influences, chronic illness, and the unique healthcare situation and context. Low health literacy has been associated with higher mortality in heart failure patients (Peterson, 2011). Assessment of health literacy begins with the initial intake or interview, using a formal tool or with observation and subjective responses from the patient such as "I don't have my glasses" or "My daughter usually fills out the forms." A nurse case manager's awareness of a patient's, family's, or caregiver's health literacy can improve self-management and adherence to the case manager plan. This is equally important when preparing case management plans, discharge instructions, and educational materials. The Institute of Medicine published guidelines for a health literate organization—*Attributes of a Health Literate Organization*—which are available at www.iom.edu. Case managers can use the following resources to design educational materials that better meet their population's needs and literacy levels:

- ▶ Case Management Adherence Guidelines: www.cmsa.org
- ▶ Center for Medicare and Medicaid Services Written Materials Toolkit (2010): www.cms.gov
- ▶ National Institutes of Health: www.nih.gov

CULTURAL INFLUENCES

Case managers, because of their key role as members of the healthcare team, have the opportunity to help ensure access to care, improve quality of care provided, and achieve positive health outcomes for patients regardless of the point of entry to the healthcare system. The increasing population growth of racial, ethnic, and linguistic groups, each with its own cultural traits and health profiles, presents a challenge to the healthcare delivery system. It is important to realize that both providers and patients bring their individual viewpoints, languages, and cultures when they meet. Attempts should be made to transcend differences in order to achieve equal access and a high-quality healthcare experience for all. According to the Office of Minority Health, culture and language may influence

- ▶ Health, healing, and wellness belief systems;
- ▶ How illness, disease, and their causes are perceived—by both the patient and the provider;

▶ The behaviors of patients who are seeking health care and their attitudes toward healthcare providers;

▶ The delivery of services by providers, who look at the world through their own limited set of values, which can compromise access for patients from other cultures (Office of Minority Health, 2010).

Healthcare professionals must have a basic understanding of the impact that language and culture have on health and healthcare delivery to effectively organize services that meet the individual needs of the population and decrease disparities that exist in our healthcare system. In this way, providers and patients can come together to talk about healthcare concerns without cultural differences hindering the conversations.

Cultural competency is key to addressing healthcare disparities. Increasingly diverse racial, ethnic, and sociocultural backgrounds of patients, families, caregivers, and colleagues affect clinical situations and healthcare outcomes. Culturally Competent Nursing Modules (CCNMs) were developed to equip nurses with the skills and knowledge to improve cultural competency. The CCNMs consist of an introduction and three modules available at https://www.ccnm. thinkculturalhealth.hhs.gov. Providing healthcare services that are respectful of and responsive to the health beliefs, practices, and cultural and linguistic needs of diverse patients can help break down barriers and ensure positive outcomes.

SHARED RESPONSIBILITY FOR LEARNING

Healthcare providers have become increasingly aware that in order to make changes in the system, they need to understand their patients and learn from data that are collected at the point of care. Case managers are professionals who are critical to the healthcare system's front lines. They determine the needs of patients, direct approaches to appropriate care, educate and empower patients, and work to ensure integrity and quality across the continuum of care. One of the advances that promises to aid in these efforts is healthcare information technology (HIT), and specifically, mobilizing health information exchange electronically. These systems, when available across the care continuum, are instrumental in assisting healthcare professionals in making significant improvements in the quality, safety, and efficiency of care.

Interoperable HIT and health information exchange, or the electronic mobilization of clinical information, facilitates access to and retrieval of clinical data, both privately and securely, by different entities involved in the care delivery system. This provides for safer, more timely, efficient, effective, and equitable patient-centered care (Institute of Medicine, 2011).

To lead the movement in incorporating these advances into mainstream health care, the Patient Protection and Affordable Care Act, enacted in March 2010, asks health plans and providers to develop electronic health records (EHRs) by 2015. Through grants and bonus payment incentives, eligible providers can offset the costs of upgrading computer infrastructure and training staff to be EHR capable. This legislation is aimed at increasing patient safety as well as the electronic exchange of health information.

Today, healthcare professionals are involved in the development and design of information technology (IT) systems that collect data at the point of care. In addition, their expertise is used to assist in the creation of innovative programs and tools, such as Integrated Care Management, that generate reports and provide evidence for healthcare decision-making—a key consideration for improving the effectiveness of medical care.

These initiatives make the collection of evidence-based healthcare data, which helps decrease variation and fragmentation, more organized and efficient. This is the result in part of the growing appreciation of the important role the patient plays in achieving positive healthcare outcomes. The sea of change emphasizes the importance for case managers and other healthcare professionals of working collaboratively with patients and of continuing to develop new technologies that expand access to timely information and evidence available at the point of care.

INTERPRETER SERVICES AND MATERIALS

To address the growing concerns about racial, ethnic, and language disparities in health, culturally and linguistic appropriate services (CLAS) have become more and more a matter of national importance. CLAS standards are defined and healthcare organizations and individual providers directed to make their practices more culturally and linguistically accessible by the Office of Minority Health (2007). The Institute of Medicine (IOM) emphasized the importance of language disparities in a report that found that those with limited English proficiency encounter significant disparities in health care, including

- ▶ Access to care,
- ▶ Being less likely to have a primary source of care,
- ▶ Receiving unnecessary diagnostic tests, and
- ▶ Serious outcomes from medical errors and drug complications (IOM, 2009b).

One way in which organizations are working to address disparities with non–English-speaking patients is through the utilization of medical interpreters and translators. A medical interpreter works with the spoken word between two languages, meaning he or she knows both languages equally well, has good communication skills, and likes working with people. A medical translator, however, works with the written word between two languages, usually translating it into his or her dominant language, rather than into the second and less well-known language. A translator has good writing and grammar skills, and is proficient with a computer and various software programs used in the translation of documents.

The Office of Minority Health sponsored the development of *A Patient-Centered Guide to Implementing Language Access Services in Healthcare Organizations* to help professionals implement effective language-assisted services that meet the needs of their limited English proficiency (LEP) patients. Case managers and other healthcare professionals can use this guide to evaluate how well their organizations are ensuring that all patients have access to safe, high-quality, evidence-based care at the right time, in the least restrictive setting in the most cost-effective manner, which is the essence of the practice of case management.

POPULATION HEALTH MANAGEMENT, WELLNESS PROMOTION, AND ILLNESS PREVENTION

DISEASE MANAGEMENT

Historically, the delivery of health care in the United States has focused most resources, treatments, and services on addressing the acute effects of chronic disease. As a result, costs have escalated and outcomes reported have not justified expenditures. Chronic disease and disability are major "drivers" of healthcare utilization and the associated costs.

Statistics from the Centers for Disease Control and Prevention (CDC) estimate that more than 90 million Americans live with chronic illness, and 7 out of 10 deaths per year are related to chronic diseases. Heart disease, cancer, and stroke account for more than 50% of all deaths each year. Worldwide, chronic diseases account for 35 million deaths per year; sub-Saharan Africa is the only part of the world where more people die from infectious diseases than chronic diseases (CDC, 2009).

Attempts to control costs are further complicated by the graying of America and numerous scientific advances that have enabled people to survive longer with complex medical conditions. Employers, payers, and government officials have demanded that the healthcare industry find a more efficient and effective method to provide healthcare services.

Pathophysiology

To help people better cope with chronic illness, nurse case managers must understand the pathophysiological and psychological aspects of the disease process so that they can encourage patients and families to make positive behavioral changes and to learn self-management skills that will allow them to more readily adapt to their conditions. When patients are empowered to self-manage, adherence to the plan of care increases, techniques are used to better manage complications, and disability is minimized.

For nurse case managers to be successful educators, they need to have a thorough understanding of the current clinical issues pertaining to a particular disease. Many managed care organizations offer disease management (DM) programs and have assigned nurse case managers to specialize in specific disease areas. Patients served by these DM programs include those with high-risk pregnancies, transplants, AIDS and AIDS-related diseases, asthma, chronic obstructive pulmonary disease, chronic heart failure, and long-term pediatric complications (e.g., those requiring neonatal care or cancer treatment). Specialization in a specific area allows the nurse case manager to develop relationships with appropriate providers and centers of excellence that offer specific treatment and service options, thereby better equipping the case manager to more effectively and efficiently meet the patient's and family's needs.

Once a person is identified as having been diagnosed with a chronic illness, a multidisciplinary team of experts constructs a proactive program to address the diverse needs of the patient. These coordinated healthcare interventions and communications use various tools such as

- ▶ Health risk assessments,
- ▶ Clinical guidelines,
- ▶ Call center triage,
- ▶ Formularies,
- ▶ Evidence-based practice, and
- ▶ Home telemonitoring.

These experts work closely with the patient's physician or nurse practitioner since he or she is legally licensed to diagnose and treat the patient and, therefore, is the most appropriate provider to determine the treatment plan. Goals of an effective DM program are improved quality of life and decreased healthcare costs.

Case Simulation: A respiratory therapist case manager monitors and educates an asthma patient who started on a new routine of using a peak flow meter. She explains that the meter, which measures lung capacity and functional levels, can help the patient better manage activities and self-adjust medications to fit his physical and functional requirements. She shows the patient how to accurately read the meter and to be cognizant of alerts to conditions that require immediate medical attention, such as an upper respiratory infection that can trigger an acute episode of wheezing. Early identification of asthma triggers allows the patient to adjust medications to control attacks. By developing a routine of regularly measuring peak flows, the patient has learned to recognize whether preventive measures are working or if he needs to seek medical attention.

The outcomes that this particular asthma disease management program can claim just through this singular proactive education are

- ▶ Improved patient and provider satisfaction,
- ▶ Improved clinical status,
- ▶ Improved functional status,
- ▶ Appropriate use of healthcare resources,
- ▶ Decreases in lost time at work or school, and
- ▶ Decreases in healthcare spending on reactive care.

Psychosocial Conditions

Chronic diseases take patients and families through periods of good health mixed with periods of sickness. Facing a chronic illness naturally leads to feelings of anger, anxiety, sadness, and a variety of emotions that can often complicate care. Depression should not be dismissed as a "normal" reaction to chronic illness, but it is common (National Alliance on Mental Illness, 2009). To support and empower patients and families to develop coping strategies, case managers must be aware that each person reacts to and handles problems in his or her own way. Listening to patients and family members talk about how they are coping is a vital skill for case managers. Understanding the impact a chronic illness or catastrophic injury has on family dynamics is also important.

Communicating the psychosocial and mental health issues that the patient, family, or caregivers experience is a vital function of the nurse case manager. The interdisciplinary team must be sensitive to the range of emotions these people experience (e.g., denial, confusion, fear, avoidance, anger, grief, guilt) and recognize that these emotions lead to behaviors that affect self-care, adherence, and ultimately, the chronic disease outcome. Providing support during these times is essential. This may entail referral to social services, guidance on how to sign up for community support groups, or recommendations for online support programs. The objective is that the patient and his or her family is aware of the various options available to them.

Cultural and Religious Influences on Disease

The United States is a melting pot of many different cultures. Nurse case managers work with patients from all walks of life. Diversity in health care refers to the variations among groups of people with respect to habits, values, preferences, beliefs, taboos, and rules for behavior determined to be appropriate for individual and societal interactions. It means not only is the person unique, but also that there may be societal gaps based on religion, gender, ethnicity, sexual orientation, age, birthplace, and many other characteristics that are responsible for strongly ingrained beliefs and values. Providing care effectively to persons from a multiplicity of cultures is called *cultural competence*. Cultural competence is defined as an ongoing evaluation of knowing, respecting, and incorporating the values of others. Healthcare professionals and patients bring their individual learned patterns of language and culture to the healthcare experience. As previously mentioned, being respectful and responsive to diverse populations' cultural beliefs can break down barriers and ensure positive healthcare outcomes.

Nurse case managers must look at each patient individually to make a cultural assessment. They also need to recognize their own cultural values in seeking cultural competence. Lack of understanding of cultural practices can result in challenges with adherence to care, longer hospital stays, and loss of meaningful communication between the patient and the nurse case manager.

Case managers also need to be cognizant of a person's spirituality. Taking the time to talk with the patient during the assessment and learning about his or her spiritual preference is an important, yet often overlooked, part of the planning process. Incorporating spirituality into the case management plan of care can help patients and the patient care team better address any healthcare challenges.

WELLNESS PROMOTION AND ILLNESS PREVENTION

The promotion of health and wellness has always been a goal of the healthcare team. Despite the fact that the healthcare infrastructure allows for the majority of care to be delivered as a reaction to injury or illness, rather than as a preventive action, society has long believed that all citizens have a fundamental right to wellness. In 1966, national legislation called the Partnership for Health Act recognized health as a state of complete physical, mental, and social well-being, not merely the absence of disease or injury (Peplau, 1974).

During the years since the tumultuous 1960s, a concept emerged that health care is more than medical care. Hildegarde Peplau, EdD, RN, professor emeritus of Rutgers, the State University of New Jersey, wrote the following in 1974 regarding the evolving theory of health care, which is still relevant today:

> It is an interdisciplinary enterprise requiring the interdigitation [integration] of knowledge from many sources and the interrelation of many different expert practices of many different independent professions. (Peplau, 1974)

In this statement, Peplau aptly described the case management process, which gathers knowledge and expertise from many sources and cultivates coordination among interdisciplinary, independent professionals to promote wellness.

Another element necessary to promote wellness and prevent illness is the recognition of the physical and psychological characteristics of wellness.

Physical Characteristics of Wellness

In order to promote wellness in patients with chronic conditions, nurse case managers have to educate patients about the importance of cause and effect. If a patient notices a subtle change in his or her condition, he or she must know how to react. Working closely with patients and educating them on how to handle problems is empowering for patients who want to take back control of their lives. One way that case managers empower patients is by encouraging them to keep records of daily activities and challenges, better enabling them to share information with healthcare providers. Such activity logs help providers recognize developing patterns and adjust the plan of care accordingly. Patients also should know which problems to report immediately, so that they can get help before a major crisis occurs.

Unfortunately, some patients are reluctant to contact their doctors or feel that if they often report problems, they will be seen as problem patients. The nurse case manager should try to dispel this fear and encourage the patient to be open and honest. The nurse case manager should also inform providers about positive events or achievements as part of managing the patient's condition. This allows the team to have the opportunity to give positive reinforcement to the patient rather than focus solely on problems.

In today's world of information technology, patients with chronic illness are able to gather information about their conditions in the privacy of their own homes and then transmit the information to nurses in call centers who monitor the data. In the case of heart failure patients, they are taught to take their own pulse, blood pressure, and weight, and to answer simple questions such as how they are feeling, whether their feet are swollen, and whether they took their medication(s) as instructed. When patients enter this information into a telemonitoring device, it is transmitted via the Internet to a central office for analysis. Red flags are programmed into the system to alert nurses if, for example, a patient's blood pressure is too high or too low, if the patient has weight gain or loss, or if the patient reports signs of shortness of breath or edema in his or her feet. Nurses with approved clinical protocols on their monitors contact the patient to discuss changes in medication, or to recommend the patient see his or her physician for further evaluation in the effort to proactively identify complications.

In addition to the physical characteristics of wellness, the nurse case manager must take into consideration the psychosocial status, culture, and religious beliefs of the patient. The following sample questions are suggested to assess psychosocial issues in wellness:

▶ What are the family dynamics?

▶ What is the patient's support system?

▶ What is the patient's perception of wellness?

▶ What is the role of the patient in the family structure?

▶ What is the patient's primary language? Education level? Work status? Spiritual affiliation?

As discussed previously, these points will differ from one patient to the next. Taking the time to understand the person holistically is the starting point for the case manager and patient, who together will embark on a journey in mastering health and well-being.

WELLNESS AND DISEASE-SPECIFIC EDUCATION

Nurse case managers are in a pivotal role to offer education to both promote wellness and address disease-specific needs to their patients, family, and caregivers. Wellness education assists in identification of risky behaviors and making changes that can prevent or limit illness and reduce injury. Disease-specific education focuses on self-management, geared toward raising awareness, and understanding of the condition. When options for aggressive care become limited, case managers are prepared to discuss end-of-life and palliative care options.

PREDICTIVE MODELING

Predictive modeling is a data-driven strategy used by healthcare agencies, physicians, managed care companies, and others interested in predicting costs, utilization, and even outcomes when specific variables are applied. Managed care organizations identify chronic conditions that affect specific populations and classify patients according to degree or type of risk. Those patients identified as high risk are assigned to nurse case managers who oversee healthcare services and educate the patient and family about how to better self-manage their care. Predictive modeling can confirm a correlation between a patient with a certain diagnosis and improved outcomes as a result of targeted outreach. It can also predict future behavior and anticipate the consequence of change. Using predictive modeling, case managers will be able to target the most actionable patients who will benefit from targeted outreach and education that improves the patients' overall health status but engages them in their own care, empowering the patients to take responsibility for their own health status (Hodgman, 2008).

REFERENCES

Centers for Disease Control and Prevention. (2009). *Chronic disease prevention and health promotion.* Retrieved from www.cdc.gov/nccdphp

Churchill, D. (2007). *Learning styles.* Retrieved from http://www.learnativity.com/learningstyles.html

Conner, M. L. (2004). *Andragogy and pedagogy.* Retrieved from www.agelesslearner.com/intros/andragogyassess.html

Conner, M. (2008). *What's your motivational style?* Retrieved from www.agelesslearner.com/assess/motivationstyle

Diniz, A. L., Schmidt, S., & Stothers, S. (2008). *How changes in health behavior are facilitated through adult education interventions.* Retrieved from www.wier.ca/~daniel_schugurens/faqs/qa12.html

Hodgman, S. B. (2008). Predictive modeling and outcomes. *Professional Case Management, 13*(1), 19–23.

Institute of Medicine. (2004). *Health literacy: A prescription to end confusion.* Retrieved from www.iom.edu/Reports/2004/Health-Literacy-A-Prescription-to-End-Confusion.aspx

Institute of Medicine. (2009a). *Identifying and preventing medication errors.* Retrieved from www.iom.edu/Activities/Quality/Medication errors.aspx

Institute of Medicine. (2009b). *Race, ethnicity, and language data: A standardization for healthcare quality improvement.* Retrieved from www.iom.edu/~/media/Files/Report%20Files/RaceEthinictyData

Institute of Medicine. (2011). *Health IT and patient safety.* Retrieved from www.iom.edu/hitsafety

Keesee, G. (2011). *Andragogy: Adult learning theory.* Retrieved from www.teachinglearningresources.pbworks.com/w/page/30310516/Andragogy-Adult%20Learner

Merriam, S., & Caffarella, R. (1999). *Learning in adulthood* (2nd ed.). San Francisco: Jossey-Bass.

National Alliance on Mental Illness. (2009). *Depression and chronic illness: Fact sheet.* Retrieved from www.nami.org/Template.cfm?Section=Depression&Template=/Content Management/ContentDisplay.cfm&ContentID=88875

Office of Minority Health. (2005). *A patient-centered guide to implementing language access services in healthcare organizations.* Retrieved from http://www.minorityhealth.hhs.gov/Assets/pdf/Checked/HC-LSIG.pdf

Office of Minority Health. (2007). *National standards on culturally and linguistically appropriate services.* Retrieved from www.minority health.hhs.gov/templates/browseaspx.?lvl=2&lvlD=15

Office of Minority Health. (2010). *What is cultural competency?* Retrieved from www.minorityhealth.hhs.gov/templates/bowse/aspx?lvl=2&lvlid=11

Peplau, H. (1974). Is healthcare a right? *Image: Journal of Nursing Scholarship, 7*(1), 4–10.

Peterson, P. (2011). Health literacy and outcomes among patients with heart failure. *JAMA, 305*(16), 1695–1701.

Prochaska, J. O., & Prochaska, J. M. (2011). *Best practices in the behavior management of disease.* Retrieved from www.samples.jbpub.com/9780763780434/80432_CH02_Final

U.S. Department of Health and Human Services. (n.d.). *Culturally competent nursing care: A cornerstone of caring.* Retrieved from https://ccnm.thinkculturalhealth.hhs.gov/

U.S. Department of Health and Human Services. (2010). *Quick guide to health literacy.* Retrieved from www.health.gov/communication/literacy/quickguide/factsliteracy

APPENDIX A

REVIEW QUESTIONS

5|5

1. Utilization management is best described as:

    a. being synonymous with case management.
    b. a forward-looking process to manage healthcare resources effectively.
    c. ensuring the "5 Rs".
    d. evaluating the cost-effectiveness and efficiency of health care.

2. Which of the following diagnoses should trigger case management services?

    a. Multiple sclerosis, traumatic brain injury, spinal cord injury
    b. Conjunctivitis, traumatic brain injury, cerebrovascular accident
    c. Cerebrovascular accident, migraine, asthma
    d. Non-Hodgkin's lymphoma, above-knee amputation, migraine

3. Case-finding, assessment, and formulating short- and long-term goals are all part of the:

    a. return-to-work assessment.
    b. precertification process.
    c. utilization management review.
    d. case management process.

4. Ongoing assessment of the case management care plan is part of which of the following processes?

    a. Goal-setting
    b. Retrospective review
    c. Monitoring and evaluation
    d. Facilitation

5. Case managers are committed to providing the patient options for care and respecting the patient's decisions. These actions illustrate which ethical principle?

    a. Autonomy
    b. Beneficence
    c. Justice
    d. Veracity

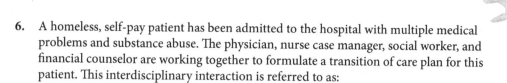

6. A homeless, self-pay patient has been admitted to the hospital with multiple medical problems and substance abuse. The physician, nurse case manager, social worker, and financial counselor are working together to formulate a transition of care plan for this patient. This interdisciplinary interaction is referred to as:

    a. collaboration.

    b. continuity.

    c. coordination.

    d. negotiation.

7. There are two basic categories of guardianship. Guardianship of:

    a. person and guardianship of health.

    b. person and guardianship of estate.

    c. health and guardianship of property.

    d. person and guardianship of trust.

8. Adult learning is an important concept nurse case managers need to consider as they educate patients about their individual conditions. Which statement best illustrates an understanding of the concept of adult learning?

    a. Children and adults have the same learning patterns.

    b. Because of nonadherence with the nutrition recommendations, the case manager closes the case because the patient obviously does not want to improve.

    c. When designing educational activities, the case manager does not use the patient's own life experience to demonstrate a point because it is not relative to the patient's new life with diabetes.

    d. The case manager involves the patient with diabetes in the care plan by having the patient keep a food diary and reviewing the diary during their weekly phone call.

9. Race, ethnicity, and language have been identified as barriers to good health outcomes. Which statement demonstrates an outcome that can be expected when language-assisted services are implemented to address disparities among impacted populations?

    a. Increased use of healthcare resources

    b. Improved quality of care, health outcomes, and health status

    c. Decreased access to care because patients would understand that payment would be required up front and not seek care

    d. Increase in accounts receivable because patients would have funding information delivered in their primary language

4|5

10. Medicare and Medicaid are public payers that cover hospital care and home health services. The difference is that

   a. Medicare is regulated by Centers for Medicare and Medicaid Services (CMS).

   b. disability is the primary criterion for Medicaid.

   c. Medicaid is a joint federal and state payer.

   d. Medicare beneficiaries must carry both parts A and B.

11. Mentoring and preceptorship are commonly used role-modeling programs to maintain the learning and professional growth of nurse case managers. They differ in that:

   a. mentoring is a long-term relationship.

   b. preceptors are usually experienced case managers who provide guidance to new case managers.

   c. both mentors and preceptors focus more on the professional objectives of the nurse case manager.

   d. preceptors use a consultative approach to assist the nurse case manager in developing broader skills and knowledge.

12. Which of the following describes benchmarking?

   a. Utilizes variance tracking

   b. Enhances clinical reimbursement

   c. Improves healthcare performance

   d. Compares similar processes and organizations, according to best practices, against leaders in a given specialty

13. When there is a question regarding a claim not meeting medical criteria, the review is turned over to:

   a. the employer's benefits division.

   b. the medical director, who makes a final decision.

   c. the second-level case manager.

   d. a third-party administrator.

14. An injured worker is receiving workers' compensation benefits. His Medicare benefits are:

   a. primary to the workers' compensation benefits.

   b. secondary to workers' compensation benefits.

   c. not applicable because the worker will lose his Medicare benefit while on workers' compensation.

   d. reduced to offset the coverage for all medical needs covered by workers' compensation benefits.

5/5

15. Accreditation serves as a symbol of excellence in healthcare industry. The value of accreditation is recognized by all stakeholders because accreditation

    a. provides transparency and accountability through nationally recognized and publicly available standards.

    b. is mandated to maintain the certificate of medical necessity.

    c. offers the assurance to a nurse case manager that quality care will be provided from an accredited provider.

    d. can be substituted for compliance with state or federal requirements.

16. Abandonment may occur in many healthcare settings and for many reasons. A nurse case manager must be knowledgeable regarding abandonment because:

    a. older adults can be placed in custodial care if their family is unable to care for them.

    b. case managers need to be familiar with their legal responsibility, state laws, and their organization's policies and procedures.

    c. abandonment is always intentional and punishable.

    d. parents dropping off their infants at a fire station can be prosecuted.

17. The Patient Self-Determination Act of 1990 is best described as:

    a. legislation that will protect your job for up to 12 weeks to care for a family member.

    b. an act that requires employers and their health insurance group plans to provide temporary extension of health benefits coverage when the employee leaves the job.

    c. legislation that requires emergency rooms to screen and provide stabilizing treatment.

    d. an act that entitles patients to advance directives.

18. Case managers recognize that conflicts of interest may occur in health care. To avoid a conflict of interest, the case manager:

    a. refers patients to the home health agency owned by the physician.

    b. uses independent, objective judgment to determine if there is an actual or potential conflict of interest.

    c. ignores all educational dinners sponsored by pharmaceutical companies.

    d. agrees to give sample medications from a physician's office to a self-pay patient.

19. Which of the following describes the Patient Protection and Affordable Care Act?

    a. The legislation will prevent free choice of a medical provider by the consumer.

    b. Under this law, health care will become more fragmented, chaotic, and complex.

    c. Sections of this healthcare reform legislation focus on care coordination, case management, and transitions of care.

    d. Every state and territory will participate in patient-centered medical home pilot projects.

4/5

20. Evidence-based practice is the integration of clinical practice with the best available evidence. A case manager's use of evidence-based practice is demonstrated by

    a. contradicting a provider's order when the order does not coincide with a standard clinical guideline.

    b. enhancing clinical effectiveness and affecting the delivery of healthcare services toward quality clinical outcomes.

    c. demanding that each discharge plan conform to the CMS core measures.

    d. agreeing with the provider that a "cookie cutter" approach does not provide an effective patient relationship.

21. Which of the following best describes integrated care management?

    a. A process of utilization review using clinical guidelines to determine level of care and length of stay

    b. An organization whose focus is on benchmarking and quality measures

    c. A comprehensive, advanced care management program that integrates all medical management functions with behavioral health to optimize clinical, financial, and quality outcomes

    d. A care coordination program that employs various disciplines to deliver a full spectrum of healthcare services

22. Case managers work in a variety of settings and empower their patients to be shared decision-makers in their health care. Common denominators, regardless of practice setting, include:

    a. facilitating optimal quality outcomes, educating patients, and patient advocacy.

    b. mandating services be provided by primary care providers, coordinating care across the healthcare continuum, and collaborating with an interdisciplinary team.

    c. empowering patients to demand high-quality care, educating caregivers on payer benefits, and negotiating out-of-network benefits.

    d. advocating for patient choice in healthcare services, educating providers on healthcare reform, and determining medical necessity based on clinical care needs.

23. Nurse case managers work diligently to make their footprints in the sands of quality management. Included in quality management processes are:

    a. benchmarking, use of subjective data, and best practice profiling.

    b. peer review, risk management, and variance tracking.

    c. Joint Commission indicators, benchmarking, and utilization review.

    d. variance tracking, cultural diversity education, and risk assessment.

24. Resource management is best defined as the process of:

    a. identifying clinical guidelines that extend the length of stay.

    b. managing the healthcare benefits.

    c. identifying, coordinating, confirming, and negotiating resources to meet the individual needs of a person.

    d. using aggregate data to identify at-risk populations.

25. Health education and health promotion programs are directly linked to the theory of:

    a. behavioral change.

    b. highest grade level achieved.

    c. economic status.

    d. social status.

26. Return on investment is a measure of the company's ability to:

    a. spend revenue captured by the utilization management program to provide dividends for shareholders.

    b. use its assets to generate additional value for patients and providers.

    c. use its assets to generate additional value for providers.

    d. use its assets to generate additional value for the organization.

27. A cost–benefit analysis is best described as a

    a. data-driven strategy to predict costs, utilization, or outcomes when specific variables are applied.

    b. process that has been improved and implemented to produce superior outcomes.

    c. net profit divided by net cost and expressed as a percentage.

    d. process that demonstrates the ratio of dollars spent to savings achieved.

28. A telemetry patient with heart failure and chronic obstructive pulmonary disease requires home oxygen. The oxygen saturation is 84% on room air, at rest, and the patient is only covered by Medicare part A. What essential education will the patient and caregiver need prior to discharge?

    a. Instruction on avoiding climbing stairs and other strenuous activities

    b. Instruction on self-pay options for the oxygen, community resources, and choosing a provider

    c. Instruction on diet and energy conservation

    d. Instruction on the home oxygen delivery and service support

4/5

29. Which of the following best describes predictive modeling?

    a. Nurse case managers contact high-risk patients with diabetes for assessment and adherence to self-management such as diet, medications, and exercise leading to improved health outcomes and cost-savings.

    b. An organization evaluates the appropriateness of care and resources prior to delivery of the services.

    c. A four-stage cyclical process used to evaluate changes implemented for quality improvement

    d. A quantitative assessment used to evaluate the benefits of various intervention strategies

30. A case manager selects a screening tool to assess the likelihood of hospital readmission in an at-risk population. The selected tool will:

    a. allow the health plan to eliminate a disease or risk factor from a specific population.

    b. evaluate the case manager interventions and eliminate costly complications.

    c. predict the frequency and duration of the inpatient admission.

    d. provide a valid method of assessing those patients experiencing healthcare disparities.

31. An elderly woman with early dementia forgets to take her medications and is losing weight because of poor nutrition. She is ambulatory, with no behavioral issues. The best level of care option would be a(n):

    a. assisted-living facility.

    b. subacute care facility.

    c. skilled nursing facility.

    d. inpatient hospice.

32. A well-designed satisfaction survey can achieve:

    a. increased referrals for the organization.

    b. a reduction in overall healthcare costs.

    c. a high response rate and capture valid, reliable, bias-free data.

    d. decreased complaints regarding billing.

33. Which of the following best describes a health maintenance organization?

    a. Members are entitled to primary care and specialty services according to income.

    b. Enrollees pay for services on a sliding scale basis.

    c. It collects a predetermined periodic payment, in advance, on behalf of each enrollee.

    d. It is a self-funded employer group using a third-party administrator.

34. A nurse case manager is developing a care plan for a medically complex patient. The care plan contains elements that are:

    a. reimbursable to the service provider.

    b. individualized to the patient and within the benefits outlined by the player.

    c. measurable and relevant to the case management interventions.

    d. difficult to change throughout the continuum of care.

35. The practice of case management is designed to ensure that health care:

    a. is based on treatment offered by experienced providers.

    b. meets the standards of individual payer organizations.

    c. is provided in the least restrictive setting.

    d. is safe.

36. Case management documentation is critical because it:

    a. provides subjective data regarding social determinants.

    b. connects the care coordination across all healthcare settings.

    c. generates data for reimbursement purposes.

    d. records interventions that were declined.

37. To avoid hospital readmission, a patient requires services at a specialty clinic. Since the services are not covered under the patient's health plan, the nurse case manager intercedes with the patient's insurance company. In this situation, the nurse case manager is acting in the role of:

    a. broker.

    b. consultant.

    c. negotiator.

    d. provider.

38. Medication errors, orders for unnecessary tests, and omission of standard procedures are classified as which type of variance?

    a. Community

    b. Operational

    c. Patient

    d. Provider

39. A patient expresses dissatisfaction with the care that she has received. The patient has chronic pain that is often severe enough to compromise independence in activities of daily living and limit social activity. When discussing these issues with the patient, the nurse case manager best facilitates the patient's empowerment by:

    a. asking what the patient wants, needs, and expects.

    b. encouraging the patient to conduct a Web search on pain management.

    c. recommending the patient change healthcare providers.

    d. suggesting the patient consider home health services.

40. In the healthcare delivery system, what is the primary goal of case management?

    a. To increase that healthcare options that an organization offers

    b. To maximize the use of community resources through the referral of clients

    c. To promote the use of advanced practice nurses

    d. To reduce the fragmentation and cost of care through care coordination

APPENDIX B

ANSWERS TO THE REVIEW QUESTIONS

1. **Correct Answer: B**. Utilization management is a forward-looking process to manage healthcare resources. It may be the "trigger" into case management; however, these processes are not synonymous.

2. **Correct Answer: A.** Chronic, complex, or catastrophic illnesses or injuries should trigger case management services.

3. **Correct Answer D**. The case management process includes assessment, planning, implementation, coordination, monitoring and evaluation, and outcomes.

4. **Correct Answer: C**. The nurse case manager monitors the plan of care on a continuing basis to ensure there is progress toward desired outcomes.

5. **Correct Answer: A**. Autonomy is the principle governing a person's right to make his or her own decisions. Patients should be encouraged to make decisions regarding their healthcare treatment, even if the decisions are difficult for healthcare providers to accept.

6. **Correct Answer: A**. Collaboration is an essential skill utilized to unite the healthcare team and design a plan of care for an individual patient.

7. **Correct Answer: D**. Guardianship is classified into two categories: guardianship of person and guardianship of trust.

8. **Correct Answer: D**. Adult learners are practical and focus on what is most useful to them. Designing education that demonstrates how information is useful to the patient will have more success than general education programs.

9. **Correct Answer: B**. Information delivered in a preferred primary language improves understanding and adherence in all aspects of care.

10. **Correct Answer: C**. Medicaid is a joint federal and state public payer program, legislated as Title 19 in 1965.

11. **Correct Answer: A**. Mentoring relationships may last months or years and be determined by the time required for the protégé to achieve his or her objectives.

12. **Correct Answer: D**. Benchmarking is a process used by healthcare organizations to evaluate aspects of their processes in relation to best practice, usually within their own industry.

13. **Correct Answer: B**. When a claim does not meet the medical criteria used, it is turned over to the medical director, who makes the final decision.

14. **Correct Answer: B**. Medicare is a secondary payer for health care related to the on-the-job injury or illness. Other illnesses or injury would be covered by Medicare.

15. **Correct Answer A**. The value of accreditation is widely recognized by all stakeholders in the healthcare arena as an alternative avenue to demonstrate compliance with state and federal regulations as well as use of current best practices as quality measures.

16. **Correct Answer B**. The nurse case manager should be familiar with laws, policies, and procedures regarding abandonment to uphold the right of the patient as well as the legal responsibility of the case manager.

17. **Correct Answer: D**: The PSDA requires many Medicare and Medicaid providers to give adults information about their rights under state laws governing advance directives.

18. **Correct Answer: B**. To avoid conflict of interest, the case manager should continually consider whether the situation is likely to interfere or appear to interfere with independent, objective judgment.

19. **Correct Answer C**. The health reform legislation contains provisions that address care coordination, shared decision-making, and transitions of care. These areas are integral to case management practice.

20. **Correct Answer B**. Evidence-based practice allows the practitioner to assess current and past research, clinical guidelines, and other information resources to differentiate between high- and low-quality findings.

21. **Correct Answer C**. Integrated care management is a comprehensive, advanced care management program that incorporates all medical management functions and behavioral health management. It goes beyond traditional case management and disease management.

22. **Correct Answer: A**. Regardless of practice setting, nurse case managers employ the case management process to coordinate, facilitate, and advocate for a patient's healthcare needs.

23. **Correct Answer: C**. Nurse case managers realize that the tools developed to assist them in quality management are data-driven. Many quality management processes exist and utilize tools that are not meant to replace clinical judgment, but are used to guide and organize treatment decisions in specific situations.

24. **Correct Answer: C**. Resource management is a goal-oriented approach that requires extensive coordination and is an integral part of each step in the case management process.

25. **Correct Answer: A**. Health education and health programs are directly linked to theories of adult education and, more specifically, to the theories of behavioral change.

26. **Correct Answer: B**. Return on investment is a measure of a company's ability to use its assets to generate additional value for patients and providers.

27. **Correct Answer: D**. Cost–benefit analysis is used to demonstrate the ratio of dollars spent to savings achieved. In case management, documentation of savings achieved as a result of case management intervention is an important outcome.

28. **Correct Answer: B**. Respiratory equipment, including home oxygen, is covered under Part B Medicare. Part B coverage includes physician's services, outpatient hospital services, and medical equipment and supplies. Without Part B coverage, a supplement policy, or secondary coverage, a patient would be self-pay and need resources to secure the needed service, equipment, or supplies.

29. **Correct Answer: A**. Predictive modeling seeks to confirm a correlation between the identification of patients with a specific conditions or diagnoses and improved outcomes resulting from targeted outreach efforts.

30. **Correct Answer: D**. Health assessment screening tools are an effective means to evaluate risk and outcomes.

31. **Correct Answer: A**. Assisted living is appropriate when a person can remain relatively independent but with some assistance to ensure safety and proper nutrition.

32. **Correct Answer: C**. A well-designed patient satisfaction survey can have a high response rate and capture reliable, valid, bias-free data.

33. **Correct Answer: C**. An HMO accepts responsibility for delivering an agreed-to set of services to and products to an enrolled group for a predetermined periodic (usually monthly) payment.

34. **Correct Answer: B**. Planning is the process by which the nurse case manager develops a patient-centered, evidence-based, interdisciplinary plan of care based on complete analysis of data.

35. **Correct Answer: C**. Case managers ensure that patients receive high-quality care in the least restrictive settings for the most cost-effective price in an organized and coordinated manner.

36. **Correct Answer: B**. Case management documentation is the thread that connects all of the complex processes of patient care coordination in all settings.

37. **Correct Answer: C**. A case manager negotiates when a needed service or product is not covered by the patient's health plan. Negotiation may be necessary to facilitate a transition of care, whether internal or external.

38. **Correct Answer: D**. Provider or clinician variances are classified as an untoward occurrence related to the professional charged with caring for the patient.

39. **Correct Answer: A**. Soliciting what the patient expects is key to successful, quality outcomes. The nurse case manager may identify essential learning needs during this assessment, plus cooperation of the patient is needed to ensure adherence with the plan of care.

40. **Correct Answer: D**. Case managers are vital healthcare professionals to reduce fragmentation of care, decrease health care silos, and promote cost-effective, high-quality outcomes.

INDEX

INDEX

ABOUT THE AUTHORS

Margaret Leonard, MS, RN-BC, FNP, is a national leader in healthcare innovation, playing a key role in all major aspects of healthcare policy and practice. Senior Vice President for Clinical Services for Hudson Health Plan (Hudson), a cutting edge not-for-profit Medicaid-managed healthcare organization in New York State, Margaret is a published author, former radio program co-host and producer, and a nationally recognized speaker who has amassed dozens of awards for research, community leadership, distinguished public health service, advocacy, and case management leadership.

Margaret co-chairs Hudson's Quality Improvement Committee, the Utilization Management, Medical Encounter Data Submission, and the Supporting Excellence Operations Committees. Recognized for leadership qualities as past president and current Public Policy Committee chair emeritus of the Case Management Society of America (CMSA), member of the National Quality Forum (NQF) Quality Measurement, Research and Improvement Council, chair of the National Transitions of Care (NTOCC) Public Policy Task Force, sits on the editorial boards of three case management publications, is a member of the New York State Board of Nursing and adjunct instructor at the College of New Rochelle, School of Nursing teaching Politics of Healthcare. She received her master's degree (magna cum laude) and post-master's certification as a family nurse practitioner from Adelphi University. Margaret knows health care from all angles.

Elaine A. Miller, MSN, RN-BC, received her BSN from the State University of New York at Plattsburgh and MSN from the University of Virginia. Her nursing practice has included oncology, nutrition support/home infusion, home health/community-based services, and physical rehabilitation. Elaine has more than 12 years of case management experience and received Nursing Case Management certification from ANCC in 2002. She is a member of the Hampton Roads and Alamo Case Management Society of America (CMSA) chapters. Elaine also serves as a member of the CMSA Education Committee and as a director with the Hampton Roads-CMSA chapter. Elaine is faculty for the Nurse Case Management reviews with the American Nurses Credentialing Center. Her publications include manuscripts in *Home Health Care Nurse, Home Health Care Advisor, Case In Point,* and *The Case Manager.* Elaine has been faculty for national, state, and regional meetings on home health care and case management topics. In 2008, she was selected for the Award of Service Excellence from the CMSA. Elaine is presently supporting our wounded service members as a Nurse Case Manager with the Naval Medical Center in Portsmouth, Virginia.

Review and Resource Manual

Nursing Case Management

Addendum to the 4th Edition

CONTINUING EDUCATION RESOURCE

NURSING CERTIFICATION REVIEW MANUAL

CLINICAL PRACTICE RESOURCE

Elaine A. Bruner, MSN, RN-BC

NURSING KNOWLEDGE CENTER

The American Nurses Credentialing Center (ANCC), a subsidiary of the American Nurses Association (ANA), provides individuals and organizations throughout the nursing profession with the resources they need to achieve practice excellence. ANCC's internationally renowned credentialing programs certify nurses in specialty practice areas; recognize healthcare organizations for promoting safe, positive work environments through the Magnet Recognition Program® and the Pathway to Excellence® Program; and accredit providers of continuing nursing education. In addition, the ANCC's Institute for Credentialing Innovation provides leading-edge information, education services, and products to support its core credentialing programs.

Contents

Introduction to the *Nursing Case Management Review & Resource Manual* Addendum

The requirements for nursing case managers and the needs of patients are constantly evolving alongside new research, techniques, policies, and technologies. The Nursing Knowledge Center recognizes the importance of staying abreast of these changes. This addendum includes information from the revised test content outline to ensure the *Nursing Case Management Review and Resource Manual* is up to date. This additional information will assist you with successful completion of the certification exam and may be used as a guideline for your practice. While this addendum highlights these content areas, it is not meant to be all-inclusive. For detailed information, we encourage you to explore the topics, using the nursing case management reference list. We hope you will find this content useful as a study guide and a source of information for your practice.

Questions regarding this addendum should be sent to revmanuals@ana.org.

CHAPTER 2

Fundamentals

NURSE CASE MANAGEMENT: ROLES AND FUNCTIONS

Clinical competency and integrated care management are vital skills in Nurse Case Management (NCM) practice. Guiding principles, to demonstrate case management practice, are outlined in the CMSA *Standards of Practice* (see p. 24 of Review and Resource Manual). These principles target patient stability, wellness, and autonomy through case management processes and functions. Using these principles produces care that is patient-centered, effective, timely, appropriate, efficient, and equitable.

BIOPSYCHOSOCIAL HEALTH

A complete and comprehensive assessment is crucial to creating the NCM plan. Beyond the patient, family, and caregiver as data sources, payers and the electronic medical record offer key inflormation to compile a holistic case management assessment. The history and physical examination offer medical and biological data. But what about immigration status? Health literacy? Spiritual preference? End-of-life wishes? The psychosocial, financial, and developmental data may drive needed resources, barrier identification, and healthcare reimbursement. The assessment is not just targeted to the patient but also the family unit and community.

Successful care transitions begin with a complete biopsychosocial assessment. Your assessment will identify those who need assistance as well as those who are not receiving adequate help. Assessment is a fluid and dynamic activity that is used consistently throughout the care continuum. Every identified barrier begins with an assessment. The NCM encounters a sudden change in clinical status, a discharge plan, or the willing and able caregiver—that requires assessment. NCM assessment data with other healthcare team input offers common data elements and standardized healthcare outcomes for a safe, seamless transition of care.

EVIDENCE-BASED PRACTICE

Yogi Berra said, "In theory, there is no difference between theory and practice. In practice, there is." Evidence-based practice (EBP) integrates clinical practice with the best available research. NCM practice is not based on outdated theories or anecdotal input. EBP is a significant process to manage quality while offering the NCM the necessary tools to enhance clinical effectiveness and impact outcomes. EBP offers the following:

- ▶ Improve the quality, appropriateness, and effectiveness of health care.
- ▶ Synthesize evidence and translate research findings.
- ▶ Integrate individual clinical expertise with best available research.

Without EBP, case managers may see:

- ▶ Inadequate care
- ▶ Variations in clinical practice
- ▶ Increase in morbidity and mortality
- ▶ Rising healthcare expenditures

LINKING PATIENT TO AVAILABLE RESOURCES

NCMs ensure that patients, their families, and caregivers have the access to resources and tools needed to manage their health conditions. The ultimate goal is self-care and management.

Assessing the patient's behavior and identifying unmet needs and barriers formulates potential resources to address these areas. Implementing and coordinating resources necessitates the following NCM skills:

- ▶ Knowledge and ability to effect change
- ▶ Critical thinking skills
- ▶ Effective communication
- ▶ Assertiveness
- ▶ Knowledge of healthcare reimbursement
- ▶ Collaboration with healthcare team and stakeholders
- ▶ Knowledge of patient's community and available services and organizations

CASE SIMULATION: Jim, a 24-year-old computer programmer, has been managing his diabetes with injectable insulin, diet, and exercise for more than 10 years. Recently, he became aware of an insulin pump that has an embedded blood glucose meter. Jim approaches his primary physician who consults with the medical home case manager (MHCM), Sue. Sue contacts Jim to discuss a change in his insulin delivery. Jim shares that he feels like his current regimen is not conducive to his lifestyle. He has joined a traveling soccer club that includes out of town games, overnight travel, and more strenuous training for 5 months of the year. In addition, Jim is planning to propose to his girlfriend of 3 years and feels that his injectable insulin mandates their lifestyle including meals and activities. Jim has been stable on the current regime but wishes to improve his management with the latest technology thereby sustaining glucose levels and decreasing diabetic complications. Sue agrees that a programmable pump with embedded glucose meter appears to meet Jim's goal. She checks his health insurance policy and learns that pumps are not a covered benefit. Sue requests Jim's self-care log with glucose readings and insulin doses, and contacts the pharmacy provider for a cost analysis on the insulin and required supplies. She compiles this data, along with statements from Jim's endocrinologist and diabetes nurse educator, to demonstrate that an insulin pump is a cost-effective alternative for the insurance carrier. Sue is confident that her complete research and data compilation will yield a successful result. She connects with the carrier's utilization review nurse case manager to initiate negotiations for coverage and presents the medical documentation plus the cost analysis. This information is sent to the carrier's medical director who agrees to review it and render a decision within 30 days. Jim is pleased to hear this possibility; he has already researched pumps with two pharmaceutical companies, looked at costs, and decided the pump that would be best for him. Sue forwards this additional data to the carrier and awaits their decision. A week later, Jim's endocrinologist reports that he received a call from the insurance carrier's medical director who asked questions about consistent insulin delivery and glucose monitoring. Sue offered the medical director recent evidence with diabetes management and offered that a pump was the best treatment for Jim given his age and active lifestyle. An authorization is issued and Jim expresses his gratitude to Sue and his healthcare team for their advocacy.

CHAPTER 3

Resource Management

LEVEL OF CARE OPTIONS

Skilled Nursing Facility

Per CMS policy, the Medicare benefit covers 100 SNF days after a 3-day hospital stay. Skilled nursing facility (SNF) days 1 through 20 have no co-pay from the Medicare beneficiary. Days 21 through 100 are covered with a co-pay from the beneficiary; in 2014, this co-pay was $152.00. The SNF co-pay can change every year and if there is a secondary, Medicare Advantage or MediGap plan, these costs may be different based on plan benefits. After 100 days of SNF care, the beneficiary assumes full cost of care. For a patient to qualify for another 100-day benefit, there must be a 60-day lapse without an in-patient admission to a hospital or SNF. There is no limit on the number of benefit periods available to a Medicare beneficiary. CMS offers several publications to patients, families, and caregivers at www.cms.gov to assist with a SNF transition of care.

Hospice

Hospice is a model of care not a location of care. The services are focused on symptom management and the emotional and spiritual well-being of the patient, family, and caregivers to offer comfort with a life-limiting condition. The Medicare Hospice benefit covers medical supplies and equipment; medications for symptom management; services from healthcare providers such as physicians, nurses, therapists, dietician, and home health aides; in-patient care for symptom management; and respite care, all related to the life-limiting condition. The beneficiary does not surrender their Medicare coverage for conditions outside of the terminal condition. For example, a hospice patient gets the flu, they see their primary provider and receive influenza medications. This encounter will be covered by the Medicare benefit unrelated to their life-limiting condition. As with any transition of care option, it is imperative that the nurse case manager be familiar with the Medicare benefit as well as other reimbursement sources. Additional resources are available from www.cms.gov, the National Association for Home

Care & Hospice, www.nahc.org, and the National Hospice and Palliative Care Organization, www.nhpco.org.

Palliative Care

Palliative care and hospice care may be referred to in the same manner; however, palliative care services are offered by an interdisciplinary team, often in acute care, extended care, or the home. There is no time frame for palliative care, unlike hospice where a physician certifies that the person has less than a 6-month life expectancy. Unlike an inclusive Medicare hospice benefit, palliative care costs are included with the acute care benefit or medical provider fee. Because there are no time limits for palliative care services, it is available to patients who want, or need, comfort at any stage of their condition, terminal or not. There is no expectation that life-prolonging interventions, such as chemotherapy or artificial nutrition, will be avoided. Coverage for palliative care programs may be available through commercial and public healthcare funding. Therefore, the NCM will explore any specific needs with the reimbursement source before initiation of care.

Respite Care

This level of care offers temporary relief to a patient's family or caregivers, planned or in an emergency, for adults and children with special needs. Respite services occur in the home, a facility, or with adult day care. Respite caregivers may be paid or volunteer in any model of these services. Medicare hospice benefits, Medicaid waivers, long-term-care insurance, and veterans' benefits may offer coverage for respite care. Additional information and respite resources may be found at the ARCH National Respite Network www.archrespite.org.

Adult Day Care

Adult day cares (ADC) are designed to offer safety, supervision, care, and companionship to seniors. These programs allow family or other caregivers to work, relax, and handle personal business knowing that their loved ones are safe and cared for. The goal of ADC is to delay or prevent institutionalization by providing alternative care, which encourages socialization and enhances self-esteem. There are two types of ADC: adult social day care and adult day health care (ADHC). Social day care provides meals, recreation, and some health-related services. ADHC offers intensive health services, such as medication administration, and therapeutic and social services for those seniors whose medical problems put them at risk for nursing home placement. ADC may be covered by Medicaid, long-term-care insurance, or self-pay. It is essential to research ADC availability as the services may vary. Area Agencies on Aging and the Eldercare Locator are excellent sources for ADC information.

PAYER AND REIMBURSEMENT METHODOLOGY

Medicare is a federally funded/public payer administered by the Centers for Medicare & Medicaid services (CMS). The Medicare entitlement has four benefits or parts:

▶ Part A-Hospital Insurance

▶ Part B-Medical Insurance

▶ Part C-Medicare Advantage Plan (managed care)

▶ Part D- Prescription Plan

Medicare eligibility is based on work contributions to Social Security through FICA tax. Individuals with the following criteria are Medicare-eligible:

▶ U.S. citizens 65 years or older

▶ Permanent legal resident for 5 continuous years and 65 or older

▶ Qualifying disability (blindness) or medical condition (Amyotrophic Lateral Sclerosis)

▶ Received SSDI for 24 months

▶ End-stage renal disease on dialysis, or received a kidney transplant

▶ A child or widow(er) age 50 or older, including a divorced widow(er), of someone who has worked and paid FTCA tax, and meets the SSDI criteria

See Chapter 3 in the *Review and Resource Manual, 4th Ed.* for additional content.

SUPPORT SERVICES

Benefits and payment for support services vary, depending on the service. Some are state-supported such as Department of Public Health, the Special Supplemental Nutrition Program for Women, Infants, and Children (WIC), and the Department for Aging and Rehabilitative Services (DARS). Others are through voluntary organizations such as the American Red Cross, American Cancer Society, or United Way. Faith-based organizations may be a resource for transportation, homemaker, and nutrition services such as a food pantry or meals. These services may be free or offered on a donation basis. Legal services may be paid on a sliding scale, fee-for-service, or may be pro bono through law schools, community agencies, or law firms. Medication assistance programs may offer prescriptions free or at a reduced fee — for example, all antibiotics for $5.00 per 10-day supply. Many pharmaceutical companies offer prescription assistance. These programs have specific criteria and guidelines for persons to qualify and are administered by each pharmaceutical company. A patient with multiple medications who qualifies for assistance may be working with several pharmaceutical companies. Community agencies such as the Area Agency on Aging or United Way may have assistance available to complete prescription assistance documentation. Finally, a long-term-care policy may cover services such as adult day care, meals, pet care, and home modifications.

NEGOTIATING FOR PROVIDERS, SUPPORT SERVICES, SUPPLIES, AND DURABLE MEDICAL EQUIPMENT

Services or products that are not covered may be offered as a contracted benefit or a carve-out. For example, Long Term Acute Care (LTAC) may not be a covered level of care yet the patient would benefit from the complex medical care plus rehabilitation which is not as available in an ICU. Persons may have needs that are a non-covered benefit which are cost-effective and provide a safe transition of care. In these circumstances, the NCM uses negotiation skills to explore possible coverage. (see previous Case Simulation in Fundamentals). Covering ADL services with a home health aide may be preferred by the patient and less expensive than custodial care. Specific durable medical equipment (DME) may reduce complications, such as decubitus ulcer, with a modified wheelchair or special cushion. It is crucial to offer a comprehensive assessment, plan, and cost savings to the potential payer to yield a favorable response.

Before a referral, it's vital to research which providers are in-network with a payer through a phone call or online data base. In-network providers may change frequently so current information is essential. Patients, families, or caregivers will need instruction on co-payments or out-of-pocket expenses before receiving the product or service.

CASE SIMULATION: It is day 46 for Mary, 58 years old, s/p left MCA stroke. She is ventilator-dependent with a tracheostomy, receives nutrition support by way of PEG, and has several IV medications. The ICU team recommends LTAC for pulmonary rehab/vent weaning as well as physical rehabilitation. Mary is able to communicate by shaking her head and occasionally writing. Her family is anxious to care for her; they visit daily and have learned passive range of motion (PROM) and active range of motion (AROM) exercises from the OT and PT providers. The NCM, Ann, gathers the medical documentation and daily cost of ICU care to present to the patient's health insurance provider. It is clear that LTAC is more cost-effective and offers Mary less complications and a bridge to continued care in an acute rehabilitation (IRF) or home care. The health plan agrees to LTAC and offers to cover 14 days, initially, with periodic updates to continue coverage. Should Mary's progress plateau, then the health plan has a skilled nursing facility (SNF) benefit. Ann communicates this plan to the ICU team and Mary's family who agree. Mary's family understands that progress must be demonstrated for the health plan to continue coverage. Both the patient and family are pleased with the transition of care. Ann contacts the chosen LTAC to initiate a referral and the family tours the facility. Transfer documentation is completed, ambulance transport is scheduled, and Ann contacts the receiving LTAC case manager with a report. After 24 hours, Ann contacts the LTAC case manager to offer additional information or clarify transfer data.

CHAPTER 4

Quality Management

CORE MEASURES

Emergency Department (ED) core measures expanded to include the following indicators:

- ▶ Use of CT scan for atraumatic headache. (2012)
- ▶ Head CT scan results for acute ischemic stroke or hemorrhagic stroke patients who received head CT scan interpretation within 45 minutes of arrival. (2013)
- ▶ Troponin results for ED acute myocardial infarction patients or chest pain patients (with probable cardiac chest pain) received within 60 minutes of arrival. (2013)
- ▶ Median time to pain management for long bone fracture. (2013)
- ▶ Patient left before being seen. (2013)
- ▶ Door to diagnostic evaluation by a qualified medical professional. (2013)
- ▶ Median time from ED arrival to ED departure for discharged patients. (2013)
- ▶ Median time from ED arrival to ED departure for admitted patients. (2014)
    - ▶ Separate reporting for observation patients and psychiatric/mental health patients.
- ▶ Admission decision time to ED departure for admitted patients. (2014)
    - ▶ Separate reporting for psychiatric/mental health patients.

These expanded measures extend throughout activities, which has resulted in increased collaboration between ED providers, hospitalists, and acute care and in-patient units. These are more than "door to doctor" metrics. Critical goals of the ED measures are to relieve crowding and improve patient satisfaction as well as to improve outcomes. In addition, the updated measures improve access to treatment and increase quality of care.

Other metrics such as the Joint Commission's Surgical Care Improvement Project (SCIP) address measures for surgical infection prevention, beta blocker therapy, and venous thromboembolism (VTE). Individual organizations and facilities have developed specific measures, dashboards, and other means of quality assurance to provide transparency to the healthcare consumer as well their stakeholders.

CHAPTER 5

Legal and Ethical Considerations

HIPAA OMNIBUS RULE—MARCH 26, 2013

The HIPAA Omnibus Rule is the final rule mandated by the Health Information Technology for Economic and Clinical Health Act (HITECH). This rule strengthens patient privacy protections and provides patients with new rights to protected health information (PHI). Covered entities and healthcare providers were required to comply by September 23, 2013. Some highlights of the omnibus final rule:

▶ It allows patients to ask for a copy of their electronic health record in electronic form.

▶ When patients pay out of pocket in full, they can instruct their provider to refrain from sharing information about their treatment with their health insurance company.

▶ If a Medicare beneficiary requests a restriction on the disclosure of PHI to Medicare for a covered service and pays out of pocket for the service, the provider must also restrict the disclosure of PHI regarding the service to Medicare.

▶ The final rule sets new limits on how information can be used and disclosed for marketing and fundraising purposes, and it prohibits the sale of a person's health information without their permission.

▶ Penalties for noncompliance with the final rule are based on the level of negligence with a maximum penalty of $1.5 million per violation.

HEALTH INFORMATION TECHNOLOGY FOR ECONOMIC AND CLINICAL HEALTH ACT — 2009

The HITECH Act widens the scope of privacy and security protection under HIPAA, increasing the potential legal liability for noncompliance and providing more enforcement. The intent is to promote adoption and meaningful use of health information technology plus strengthen the civil and criminal enforcement of HIPAA.

PATIENT PROTECTION AND AFFORDABLE CARE ACT

Under Title III, accountable care organizations (ACO) were created from the Affordable Care Act (ACA) in the belief that they will improve healthcare quality and decrease healthcare spending. An ACO is defined as a collection of healthcare providers — primary care, hospitals, and specialists — who work collaboratively and accept collective accountability for the cost and quality of care delivered to a group of patients. Because the ACO includes many primary care providers, medical practices, and specialists, it can be thought of as a "medical neighborhood." To be successful, the ACO must have seamless information sharing, which means an integrated IT system. This care delivery re-design aims to improve efficiency and quality plus offer cost containment across the healthcare continuum. Cost savings result from coordinated, less fragmented, and duplicated care. According the Kaiser Health News, 14% of Americans are enrolled in an ACO.

COLLABORATING AND ADVOCATING FOR ACCESS TO CARE

In the United States the greatest barrier to access to care is lack of health insurance. The ACA has offered millions of Americans coverage under Medicaid and the federal or state health exchanges. Even with coverage, access to care may have barriers such as complex medical problems or mental health issues. For the medically complex patient, a proactive approach to anticipate care and services as well as exploring alternatives offers collaboration among the healthcare team as well as stakeholders. Until there is a true parity for mental health care vs. physical health care, there will be a need for consistent advocacy to achieve appropriate care, safe transitions, continuing services, and quality outcomes. Persons who need unfunded or underfunded services face multiple challenges and choices regarding health care. The individual mandate under the ACA states that everyone has a health plan, either public or private payer. However, people will choose to remain unfunded when faced with meeting basic expenses such as food and clothing. This population will need a variety of resources and a champion for their healthcare needs. The NCM fits this need by offering expanded knowledge and tools with which to advocate for the self-pay or underfunded patient.

CHAPTER 6

Education and Health Promotion

MOTIVATIONAL INTERVIEWING

Motivational Interviewing (MI) is a collaborative, person-centered, and evidence-based form of guiding to elicit and strengthen motivation for change. MI was first reported in 2002 as an intervention for addiction treatment. It is a treatment that can address ambivalence to change. Techniques used in MI are nonjudgmental, non-confrontational, and non-adversarial. As a nurse case manager, you want to be persuasive not coercive. Our goal is not to tell a patient what to do but rather be a partner in the change process. The change arises from their internal motivation. It is a conversational approach that assists the patient in identifying possibilities and using their internal and external coping strategies to enhance adherence to their care plan.

Principles of Motivational Interviewing

EXPRESS EMPATHY

- ▶ Acceptance enhances self-esteem.
- ▶ Participant ambivalence is normal.
- ▶ Reflective listening is fundamental.

AVOID ARGUMENTS

- ▶ Change must be negotiated, not dictated.
- ▶ Coercion will not produce change and adherence to plan of care.

DEVELOP DISCREPANCY

- ▶ Change is motivated by a perceived discrepancy between current behavior and personal goals and core values.
- ▶ Discrepancy enables the patient to see that the present situation does not fit with future goals.

Roll with Resistance

- ▶ Allows the patient to explore their views.
- ▶ New perspectives are offered not imposed.
- ▶ Resistance is a signal for the case manager to offer alternative responses.

Support Self-efficacy

- ▶ Belief in the possibility of change is an important motivator.
- ▶ The patient is responsible for choosing and acting on the change.
- ▶ Likelihood of change occurring increases with the patient's belief that they have the ability to change.

(Miller & Rollnick 2002)

MI uses the concept of *elicit, provide, elicit* which offers a continuous process of communication and information exchange between the nurse case manager and the patient. Open-ended questions *elicit* a patient's attitudes, beliefs, values, and their readiness to change. Reflective listening skills are critical as they build a collaborative relationship, establish empathy, and offer clarification when needed.

Providing information addresses gaps in knowledge; it may be helpful to ask permission from the patient as this increases acceptance and decreases the impression that information is being imposed.

Once the patient has been presented with new information, the NCM *elicits* information on the patient's comprehension and their reaction about it. This approach identifies concerns or questions while allowing the patient to explain the content in their own words.

Promoting patient adherence through empathetic coaching, and focusing on patient-centered care improves clinical outcomes and enhances patient satisfaction. Motivational interviewing is an essential tool for nurse case managers as we strive to engage patients in their healthcare services.

SELECTING EDUCATIONAL MATERIALS: PROVIDING PATIENT-FOCUSED INSTRUCTION AND EVALUATING EDUCATIONAL OUTCOMES

As previously noted, NCMs assist diverse populations to attain maximum wellness and manage their illnesses or injuries. How do you choose an educational method or materials? Which teaching approach would be most effective? What outcomes demonstrate that learning or a behavior change has occurred? There is no cookie cutter method to patient education. Case managers recognize that persons bring their experiences to changes in self-management. In addition, relevance and an individual's need for new knowledge impact decisions on changing current behaviors. The following case simulation illustrates this content and considers the impact that NCMs have on a person's self-care.

CASE SIMULATION: Kay is a 38-year-old mother of three teenagers and her husband, Bob, is deployed with his Marine Command. She works in a part-time position as a realtor. Recently, Kay was discharged from the ED after an episode of dizziness and nausea. Discharge diagnosis is essential hypertension (HTN). Discharge instructions are to see her PCP within 2 weeks, begin HTN medications as instructed, and adhere to diet recommendations with low sodium. The NCM with her PCP meets Kay during her follow-up appointment for disease management education. B/P=156/92.

NCM: How do you feel about taking HTN medication and adapting to a low salt diet for your high blood pressure?

Kay: It's been hard to remember the medicine plus I don't feel like it's working; I don't feel any different. And the low salt foods are bland plus I'm too busy with the kids. I shuttle them to activities 5 days a week. My youngest son has tutoring after school 3 days a week and the older two are in soccer. It's exhausting. Then we still have homework to do when we get home at 7 P.M. My phone and iPad schedules are full each day with appointments, errands, and the boy's activities.

NCM: Sounds like you and your family are busy during the week. What could help you remember your HTN medicine?

Kay: Why should I keep taking it if I don't feel any effects?

NCM: I hear that you don't feel any effect from the new medicine. How important do you think it is to treat your high blood pressure?

Kay: I guess I should pay more attention to caring for myself. It's only me with the boys. Do you have any idea how crazy every day is at my house? Bob will be back in 6 months. Some days that feels like forever even though our family has been through several separations and deployments. I thought it would get easier when the boys got older. Anyway, I can't be out of commission with getting sick.

NCM: You say you know you should take care of yourself. What do you think would help?

Kay: I barely remember lipstick. I don't know how I can be better with the low-salt diet and remembering the pills.

NCM: Well, I have some thoughts on what could help. May I share them and you can tell me what would work for you?

Kay: Okay. I know I need to do better. My husband said I look exhausted.

NCM: There are two apps that you can use to help plan meals that I'd like you to check out. One is for fast food and the other is for grocery shopping. It has ideas on other flavors or spices to substitute for salt. This app also helps you read food labels because sodium or salt can be hidden in many ingredients.

Kay: Well, I never go anywhere without my phone or iPad so I could load these apps then use them when we go to the fast food drive-thru before soccer. Shopping has become more difficult. Can I have this soup? What about this cheese? So, can the app you mentioned tell me those answers?

NCM: It sure can. And if you have a shopping list, then load it and you just move between the list and the app.

Kay: Something has to change so I will try these apps. Now I have to remember that pill.

NCM: How do you remember other tasks or appointments?

Kay: My calendar and agenda on my phone.

NCM: How about treating your medicine like an appointment? Set the time in your calendar with an alert.

Kay: Of course, then I can grab my coffee and get out the door. I'll put the pill bottle near my coffee mugs.

NCM: Great idea! You have created a plan to be better about your diet and medicine. How about I message/email you in a week to hear how your plan is going?

Kay: A text is the best way. I've become really proficient at it. The boys will not answer their phones—just text.

NCM: OK; we have a plan in place. Kay, I believe that you will do well. You realize you need to care for yourself and your sons. I'll get with you in a week to hear the good news. Good Luck!

One week later by text message:

NCM: Kay, this is Elaine, the Nurse Case Manager. Tell me how you are doing with your diet and pills.

Kay: Hi, I am at a soccer tournament. The pills are going Okay. A couple of days, I forgot to get coffee so I missed the pills. Then my oldest boy notices I don't have my mug when we get to school, and comments that I must have forgotten my pill, too. He is too smart and notices everything.

NCM: Everyone misses pills. Sounds like your son wants you to take care of yourself, too.

Kay: Yeah, he says he has to be the "man of the house" since his dad is deployed. He's only 12. Bob told him to take care of Mom. We skyped early this morning, and my son told on me about my pills. Bob was proud of him and really wants me to be better about caring for myself.

NCM: 12-year-olds are pretty sharp. I'm pleased to hear that he is noticing your new routine.

Kay: True. Oh, that fast food app is awesome! I can pull in and choose several meals to know which has fewer calories, fat, and salt. I have a grilled chicken sandwich right now—it's pretty tasty and a nice change from a burger.

NCM: Success! You can do this, Kay. You'll receive regular messages from me plus I'll see you at your next MD appt. in 6 weeks. We will stay in touch for questions and other information. Hope your sons win the game.

The preceding scenario illustrates several key areas in patient education and producing the desired outcome. Without arguing, blaming, or telling Kay what to do, the NCM enhanced her motivation, offered input to Kay's suggestions, then affirmed Kay's self-care. The NCM became a partner in Kay's behavior change and used the following tools:

- ▶ Motivational Interviewing
- ▶ Patient-centered education and resources
- ▶ Family support
- ▶ Acknowledging behavior change and affirming success

By acknowledging the barriers to success, the NCM expressed empathy then offered technology as the educational approach. Written materials, even online resources, may not have been appealing to Kay given her busy schedule and family responsibilities. By offering apps, Kay can receive critical information that results in the desired behavior, i.e., diet adherence.

DISEASE MANAGEMENT (ADDITIONAL TO P. 203)

As a nation, we spend 86% of our healthcare dollars on the treatment of chronic diseases. These persistent conditions—the nation's leading causes of death and disability—leave in their wake deaths that could have been prevented, lifelong disability, compromised quality of life, and burgeoning healthcare costs. (CDC, 2014). Nurse case managers have a critical role in identifying persons with high cost, high frequency chronic diseases then stratifying specific populations who are at a certain level of risk for exacerbations and hospital readmissions. CDC statistics reveal that about half of all adults—117 million people—have one or more chronic health conditions.

Seventy-five percent of Medicare readmissions within 30 days were potentially preventable, representing $12 billion in Medicare spending (MedPAC, 2014). Planning a transition of care that includes a safe, appropriate, seamless transfer from hospital to the next level of care, requires considering many elements, barriers, and opportunities. A person's biopsychosocial characteristics impact a transition of care in ways that a nurse case manager may not be able to control. Language, ethnicity, and level of education are examples of those characteristics. Hospital readmissions may be related to biopsychosocial characteristics as well as access to a primary provider, ability to pay for medications, and comprehension of the acute care discharge plan. Early identification of potential barriers, continuing care services, and caregiver support offers data which may decrease hospital readmission.

Financial incentives legislated in the Patient Protection and Affordable Care Act (2010), and penalties for readmissions, within 30 days, for Acute Myocardial Infarction (AMI), Congestive Heart Failure (CHF), and Pneumonia (PN) were effective as of October 1, 2012. In FCY 2014, CMS included an algorithm to accommodate planned readmissions for AMI, CHF and PN. Penalties for readmissions, within 30 days, were expanded in FY 2015 to include chronic obstructive pulmonary disease (COPD), total hip arthroplasty (THA), and total knee arthroplasty (TKA). The readmission data is transparent to the public and all stakeholders. Hospitals have a process to review their readmission data and submit corrections before their public release (CMMS, 2014).

POPULATION SCREENINGS

Population screenings offer early disease detection and health promotion activities. The World Health Organization (WHO) offers a tremendous amount of information on screening, detection, and surveillance for a wide range of conditions and diseases including infectious disease, non-communicable disease, injury and violence, women and health, as well as substance abuse and mental health. Screenings determine opportunities for health maintenance, wellness promotion, and symptom management. Understanding the person in a holistic manner is a pivotal starting point, which leads to the patient and nurse case manager forming a partnership to improve quality of life, wellness, and decreased healthcare costs.

References

Centers for Disease Control and Prevention (2014). *Chronic disease prevention and health promotion.* Retrieved November 27, 2014, from www.cdc.gov.nccdphp.

Centers for Medicare and Medicaid Services (2014). Retrieved November 24, 2014, from www.medicare.gov.

Centers for Medicare and Medicaid Services (2014). *Readmissions reduction program (HRRP).* Retrieved November 27, 2014, from www.cms.gov/Medicare/Medicare-Fee-for-Service-Payment/AcuteInpatientPPS/Readmissions-Reduction-Program.html.

Gold, J. (2014, April 16). FAQ On ACOs: Accountable Care Organizations, Explained. *Kaiser Health News.* Retrieved November 24, 2014, from http://kaiserhealthnews.org/news/aco-accountable-care-organization-faq/

Medicare Payment Advisory Commission (MedPAC) (2014). Retrieved from www.medpac.gov/documents/reports/mar14_entirereport.pdf?sfvrsn=0.

Miller, R. H. & Rollnick, S. (2002). *Motivational interviewing: Preparing people for change (2nd ed.).* New York, NY: Guilford Press.

World Health Organization (WHO). Retrieved November 27, 2014, from http://www.who.int/en/.